Lean Body Smart Life

12-Fix Plan to a Leaner, Healthier, Happier Life

Judith Scharman Draughon, MS, RDN, LD

Nutrition Educational Solutions, LLC

Mimi,
To a heathier life!
Judith Draughon

Copyright

This book presents the ideas of the author and is not intended to substitute for a person consultation with a health care professional. If you have any special medical conditions consult with your health care professional before starting the program contained in the book regarding possible modification for yourself. The ideas, procedures, and suggestions contained in this book are not intended as a substitute for consulting with your physician. All matters require individual medical supervision. The author shall not be liable or responsible for any loss or damage allegedly arising from any information or suggestion in the book.

The author is not responsible for your health or allergy needs that may require medical supervision. The publisher is not responsible for any adverse reaction to the recipes contained in this book.

For information about special discounts available for bulk purchases, sales promotions, fund-raising and educational needs, contact publisher or author via email.

Published by Nutrition Educational Solutions, LLC
judes@foodswithjudes.com

Table of Contents

Table of Contents

Acknowledgments

Thanks to my sweet young adult children for enjoying my recipes through the years, appreciating quality food, and supporting me in this project! Thanks to my supportive new husband for his willingness to adopt a new lifestyle and to welcome the many benefits for his life. I'm grateful to work with such a phenomenally caring person and skilled professional as Traci Fisher! Her input and willingness to collaborate have been immeasurable in completing this program. Thanks to all the dear people in my life, both personally and professionally, that encourage me and excitedly sample my food!

Introduction

The True Cost of Food

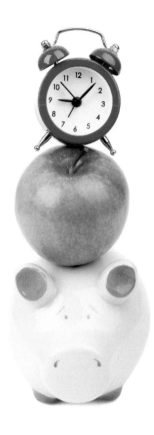

We're All in a Hurry

I want to show you how simple and fast healthy meals can be. I want to arm you with easy meal ideas so you will know just what to grab and make as you are hurrying through the grocery store trying to figure out what you can get on the table ASAP.

I want you to experience how good you can feel after eating like this for a while. You may feel so good, in fact, that you won't be lured back into eating processed convenience snacks and meals very often. You'll be disappointed when you end up stuck eating junk on the rare occasion that no other options are available. And you may even notice a lower energy and concentration level than usual on those occasions.

Delicious, Fun, and Easy

I want to show you how to eat nutrition-packed food without spending an arm and a leg—how to spend your money buying valuable nutrients that your brain and body thrive on instead of empty, low-nutrient foods that keep you foggy, tired, and craving more.

I want to reveal the mystery of processed, packaged foods once and for all. I want you to know why eating sugar and refined carbohydrates such as white flour causes your fat cells to store those calories rather than burn them. I want you to know why you crave these processed foods so you can avoid them.

No one needs to be miserable while eating nourishing, disease-preventing food. Healthy food can be delicious, fun, and easy. In fact, from the big-picture perspective, you can't afford not to eat food that is good for you.

Healthy food can be delicious, fun, and easy. In fact, from the big-picture perspective, you can't afford not to eat food that is good for you.

99

Fueling a Smarter Life

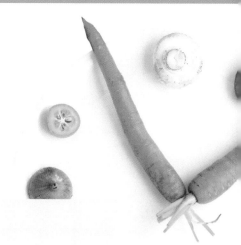

I also want people to know that the food and drinks we consume directly affect the brain's ability to function.

We don't often think of our meals and snacks as helping us accomplish our to-do lists, and yet our ability to concentrate and be productive can be slowed down by our fuel choices.

 ## Think About It.

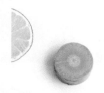

If a particular type of gas made your car move at a maximum of twenty miles per hour, you would be sure to fill your tank with a different brand that allowed you to travel at the car's maximum ability and efficiency.

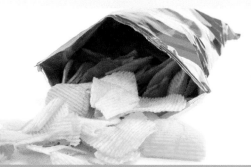

This is also true of the fuel we put into our bodies: a poor decision for lunch can truly derail an entire afternoon of productivity.

 ## Did You Know?

The average American puts on about a pound of weight every year. That might not sound like a lot, but it adds up over time. Additionally, we often lose calorie-burning muscle mass as we age. The combination of excess weight and muscle loss takes a serious toll on our figures, but worse, it makes our bodies sick and our minds dull without us even realizing what's happening.

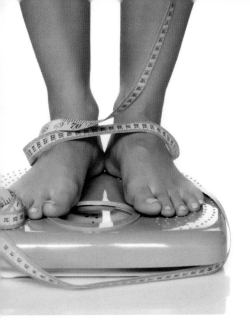

The Silent, Chronic Inflammation

Whether or not we're overweight, many of the lifestyle choices we make each day are killing us. Poor diet, activity levels, and sleep choices trigger autoimmune responses from the body, which then tries to repair itself.

Our day-after-day naive lifestyle preferences also create this constant need for the immune system to jump into action. As this cycle continues for months and then years inside our bodies, a low-grade burning, irritating effect causes damaging inflammation. This chronic inflammation is silent, so we are not aware that over time, the entire body is negatively affected by the small choices we make each day.

This long-term inflammation slowly damages our organs and our ability to function at an optimal level. It traps cholesterol, causing it to build up and make our arteries hard and rigid. I heard a heart surgeon describe this inflammation as red, angry, practically bleeding vessels that look as if the arteries had been scrubbed with a stiff metal brush several times a day.

This silent inflammation also causes insulin resistance, forcing the body to produce more insulin to balance itself. That, in turn, directs the calories we consume to be used to grow more fat cells, rather than being burned by the body for energy, making it even easier to gain more body fat and lose health-promoting muscle.

Even those without a weight issue often suffer from the ravages of insulin resistance and chronic inflammation due to diet choices and lack of exercise. All this ongoing irritation leads to rapid aging and diseases that kill both overweight and thin people. In 2013, these conditions and diseases accounted for about 75 percent of the total health-care costs. Heart disease, type 2 diabetes, cancer, Alzheimer's disease, metabolic syndrome, and sarcopenia (age-related muscle loss) are all common effects of this inflammation cycle that hurt our productivity and sabotage our quality of life.

Newer research has found that particular food patterns and exercise can lessen some of this damaging inflammation and help us improve our body composition. For those carrying excess body fat, decreasing body fat is the biggest bang for your buck. "The most powerful way to reduce your inflammatory factors is to lose excess weight," said Walter Willett, the chairman of the nutrition department at the Harvard School of Public Health.

For those who are not overweight, those same eating and movement changes needed to help lose weight can make a difference as well.

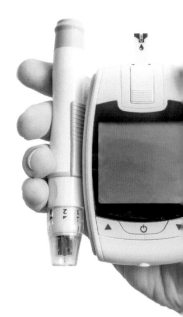

A Practical Approach to a Healthier You

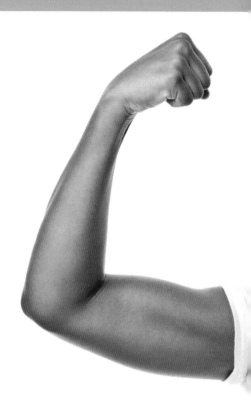

Improving Your Health Is Easy

Making a lasting weight change is a tough hurdle for many people. Every time we try to stick to a new lifestyle plan, our all-or-nothing dieting mentality sabotages us.

We get so discouraged that we end up not making any real, lasting changes.

But the truth is that losing fat and building muscle don't have to be difficult. You don't need to be on a rigid diet to see real results. You don't need to guilt-trip yourself every time you don't eat well.

In fact, the sooner you throw those fears and guilty feelings out the window, the better.

Losing weight and improving your health are easier than you think. We all make small choices that we don't realize have an impact on our health over time. The life plan in this book will identify the simple steps and attainable habits that will make the biggest impact on your weight and health using the least amount of effort.

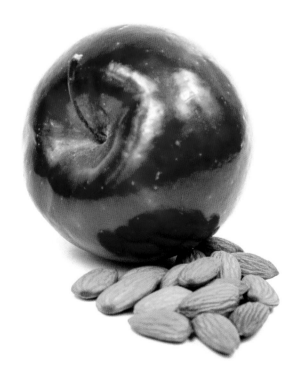

And when I say "simple," I really mean it. If you can keep unhealthy food out of sight, grab an apple, and toss a handful of almonds in a Ziploc bag before you leave for work in the morning, you have what it takes to reach your weight-loss goals.

Think About It.

Studies indicate—and I strongly believe—that doing something, however small, is better than doing nothing. I've seen this time and time again in my years of practice. Making small changes over a long period of time can make a huge difference in your health and in your life. In fact, small changes actually make a bigger difference in the long run than big changes do over a short period of time.

My plan isn't about being perfect. Any one step is designed to break the all-or-nothing dieting cycle that leaves you feeling tortured and discouraged.

You Can Feel Better

You can be healthier with fewer medical bills. You can maintain a stronger, leaner body. You can have more energy and a better quality of life to more fully enjoy your loved ones for a longer time. You can concentrate better and become more productive and successful. And you can embrace every day with the powerful knowledge that you are achieving the real changes you need to live a smarter life—physically, cognitively, and financially.

You can have all of this and more with the simplified plan I'm about to share with you, based on the latest scientific research.

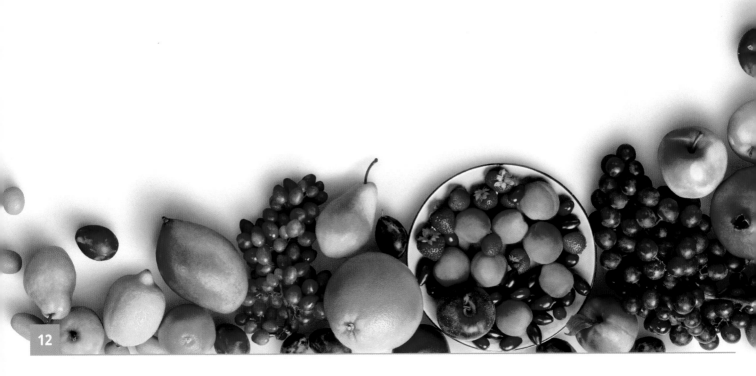

My Journey

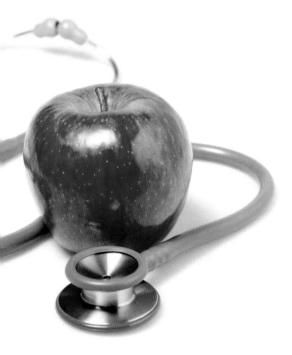

Staying On The Frontlines of Nutrition

My passion for nutrition started with a healthy love of food. In junior high school, I ran track and I wanted to know the types of foods that would help me to become the best possible runner. This interest grew over time, and in college I graduated with a Bachelor's of Science in medical dietetics, followed by a master's degree in health education. After graduate school, I traveled internationally, immersing myself in culinary cultures.

66

...I graduated with a Bachelor's of Science in medical dietetics, followed by a master's degree in health education.

99

However, what really opened my eyes to the importance of this type of work were the effects that my healthy suggestions and practices had on the real people I worked with each day. And what drove me to stay on the front lines of nutrition were the people we didn't know how to help.

I remember one client in particular: Cheryl. She came to me in 1988, when I was an outpatient dietitian at Lawrence + Memorial Hospital in Connecticut. She was confident and ambitious, and she was used to achieving her goals—but she was having trouble with her weight. Cheryl was a typical yo-yo dieter. At the time she came to see me, she was eating only about thirteen hundred calories per day, but her weight wasn't improving.

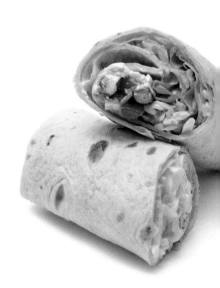

Today, we're more aware of why repetitive dieters gain back more weight than they initially lose. We are also beginning to understand that the type of calories we eat is much more important than the number of calories.

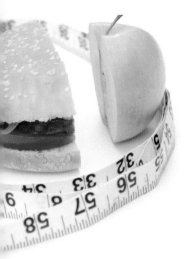

In 1988, I didn't know how to help Cheryl, and that frustrated me. I spent the next two and a half decades on my quest to find the answers that would help Cheryl and others like her.

My mission to help clients who had lost hope ultimately paid off.

As science advanced and provided us with new knowledge about weight loss, I was listening for it. Today, I continue to keep up with the latest research on nutrition. If Cheryl came to me now, I'd know exactly how to help her, and I've helped plenty of others like her over the years—by finding easy, desirable, and delicious food solutions to their health challenges.

The value of simple, healthy life changes doesn't stop at the physical level. The fixes in this book have the power to affect everything that matters as the years go by. I love the feeling of making a real, positive difference in people's lives today as much as I did back then. I thrive on helping others to make the changes they need to solve their health challenges—and oftentimes these changes don't even have to be big ones.

66

I thrive on helping others to make
the changes they need to solve
their health challenges.

99

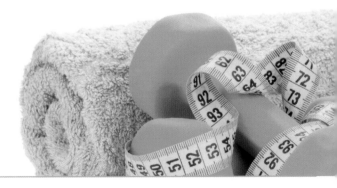

Less Is More

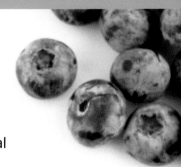

For more than twenty-five years, I've worked with thousands of people to improve their eating habits. I've spoken to many corporations, and I've helped people change their health for the better. I'm the president and founder of Nutrition Educational Solutions, more commonly known as Foods with Judes, a company dedicated to wellness. I'm also the corporate wellness dietitian nutritionist at Total Customized Fitness.

In 2010, I became an instructor at the International Culinary Arts and Science Institute. There, I educated a new generation of chefs about nutrition, and I researched new ways to make healthy foods easy, desirable, and delicious. For nine years before that, I was the president of Health and Nutrition Education Services, where I brought interactive wellness tools to thousands of children and their families.

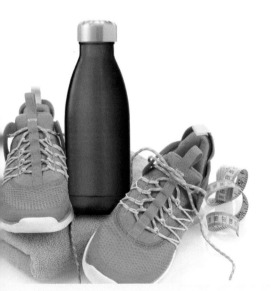

Weight Loss and Healthy Living

What is equally important is that I practice what I preach. I've spent almost thirty years unlocking the keys to weight loss and healthy living. During that time, I've been observing, studying, and investigating legitimate research on the subjects in this book. I love learning about the science behind the work. Even more, I love converting that science into easy-to-adopt practices that create a difference within the reality of daily life.

 # Think About It.

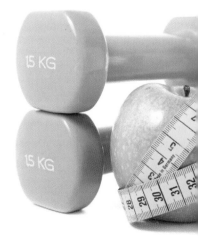

No matter who you are or what your diet history is, you can change your health for the better. I've seen it happen over and over again in my career. The small, simple steps are what make the real differences in the long run. Making some changes most of the time for the rest of your life is much better than making lots of changes for a short time.

Less truly is more!

Start with One Fix

My philosophy is simple: identify the most helpful actions to improve health and make them easier for everyone to adopt.

I've pinpointed the twelve most important actions to get the biggest bang for your effort. These behaviors are simple, sometimes seemingly insignificant, and often these behavior shifts aren't difficult when taken on individually. However, their effects can be enormous, especially when even a few of them are added together over a lifetime.

Fixes

I have a term that I will use in this book to refer to these little changes. I call them "fixes."

The twelve fixes found throughout these pages may indeed look simple, but their effects are incredibly far reaching. After just a couple of months of utilizing these fixes, you'll begin to feel more energized, awake, and astute. Your body mass will begin to shift from fat to more lean tissue. Inches will vanish from your waistline. You'll be less hungry. And as the unhealthy body fat melts away, you'll feel like you can conquer the world.

Collectively, these twelve fixes become a life plan. This 12-FIX LEAN LIFE PLAN is not like traditional weight-loss programs. It involves eating, not starving. It boosts your metabolism, rather than slowing it down. It helps fat cells burn calories, not store them.

> **This 12-FIX LEAN LIFE PLAN is not like traditional weight-loss programs.**

My 12-FIX LEAN LIFE PLAN means simple changes to your environment rather than a fight with your willpower. This plan provides action steps and research-based strategies to make healthy living easier. It celebrates successes instead of dwelling on failures. It fits into just about any lifestyle or diet restriction. This plan turns seemingly huge challenges into easy-to-reach goals.

This 12-FIX LEAN LIFE PLAN can transform your health for the better and makes it easy for you to keep it that way.

 Think About It.

Scrap the mentality that you have to do it all. This is not a diet. Any one thing that you do will help you to achieve significant results in the long term. If you exercise for one minute, that's better than zero minutes. If you eat one apple instead of a second piece of chocolate cake, that apple will do its part to reduce your inflammation, especially as new habits form.

These Fixes Are Not Difficult

It's not hard to keep less-healthy food out of sight and keep an apple on your desk at work. It's easy to change the order or the times o day you eat rather than going hungry. You will be surprised at how simple these fixes are if you concentrate on making changes one a a time, most of the time.

Track the things you do right, not the things you do wrong. Before you know it, guilt will disappear. Health and success will take its place.

> **"**
>
> Track the things you do right, not the things you do wrong.
>
> **"**

"Everything" might sound impossible, but "something" almost never is—and even if a change is small, it will bring a healthy transformation to your body over time.

When working toward a new lifestyle starts to feel overwhelming, remember: just start with one fix.

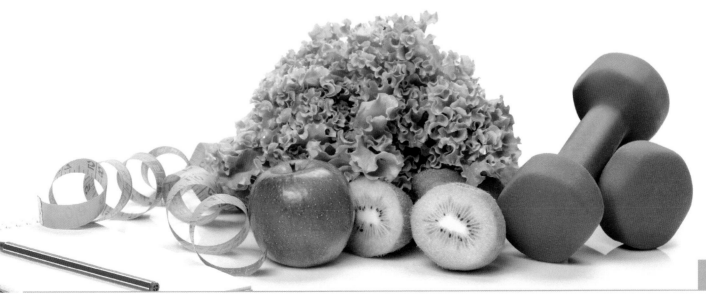

Chapter 1: Before Your Food

The New Food Paradigm: MyPlate

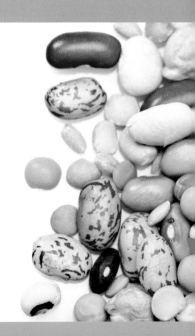

It's official: the food pyramid is history. The US Department of Agriculture's MyPlate is its new replacement, and it has big implications for your health.

With MyPlate, almost half of your meal is fruits and vegetables. That's a big change from the old model, where pasta and rice types of carbohydrates were the base of the diet. Meats have been renamed "the protein group," and the emphasis is no longer on meat. Instead, the focus is on lean, plant-based proteins such as beans, lentils, and nuts, as well as seafood containing super-healthy fat. Grains fill just over a quarter of MyPlate, and at least half of those should be whole grains. Finally, dairy is included as a side dish, such as yogurt. The next version of MyPlate will likely include water.

Did You Know?

That's a good direction for a country where only one out of four Americans eats enough fruits and vegetables. Our society as a whole suffers from obesity, insulin resistance, and silent, ongoing inflammation—irritated, red, and swollen vessels that look like they have been scrubbed with a stiff brush over and over again inside our bodies.

That's just the start. We don't get enough sleep or exercise. Heart disease, stroke, cancer, diabetes, and other illnesses kill thousands of Americans every single year.

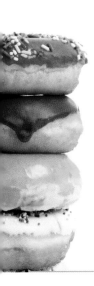

Processed Foods Epidemic

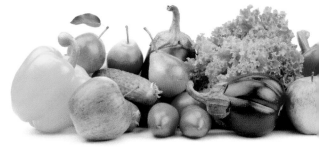

We're caught in a processed foods epidemic. With the perfect taste formula, or "bliss point," to make processed food taste additively good without costing much, packaged food products flourish. When we eat these foods, we sacrifice our health. We flood our bodies with additives, artificial colors and flavors, high-fructose corn syrup, sugar, refined white flour, salt, and less-healthy fats. We take in tons of low-nutrient processed foods that put our fat cells in grow and lockdown mode rather than burn mode.

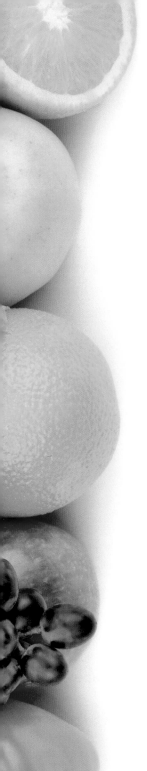

Calories from processed carbs are more likely to be used for building fat cells rather than being used as energy to function. Because these calories are locked in the fat cells and unavailable to be burned for energy, our bodies need food for energy as if we haven't eaten. Consequently, we're hungry and craving more processed carbohydrates to continue this cycle.

We make ourselves sluggish, overweight, unhappy, and sick.

But we have the power to change all that. The most powerful tools for our health aren't supplements and vitamins created in labs. They aren't new diets that take the country by storm one day and vanish the next.

The Most Powerful Tools to Improve Your Health

- Eating food in its whole form—fruits, vegetables, whole grains, plant-based proteins, fermented foods full of healthy microbes, sustainable seafood, and healthy fats, all in proportions similar to MyPlate

- Knowing what time of day to eat these foods and when to stop eating

- Drinking water throughout the day to keep your fat cells hydrated to burn more efficiently

- Moving more every day and getting a full night's sleep

- Rearranging your surroundings to replace less-helpful habits with health-promoting ones

- Losing the sabotaging all-or-nothing dieting mentality that causes you to focus on following a health plan perfectly but make you get discouraged and crash with a few mistakes.

Everything you need to begin building a healthy life is right here in this book. I'll show you how to get started.

Weight Versus Fat

This book isn't really about weight loss. It's about fat loss and becoming stronger.

The number you see on the scale doesn't mean what you think it means. It doesn't differentiate among muscle mass, water weight, and fat stores. All three of those are very different kinds of weight with very different implications for your health.

What really matters to your looks and health is how much body fat and lean tissue you have. When you lose weight, you want to lose the weight that comes from fat. At the same time, you actually want to gain weight by adding to your muscles.

Muscle plays a big role in your overall health. It appears evident from newer research that lean tissue strength greatly affects our quality of life, how well we move, and how long we live.

 Did You Know?

Starting between the ages of twenty-five and thirty, you lose a little bit of muscle every year. That adds up faster than you think. If you don't do anything to counteract it, then by the time you turn seventy-five, you've lost a lot of your natural strength. You may have trouble accomplishing basic tasks, such as twisting the lid off a jar or getting up from the couch.

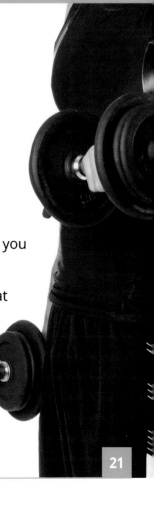

What really matters to your looks and health is how much body fat and lean tissue you have.

Increasing Muscle Mass

Muscle also helps you burn fat—even when you're not using it. The more muscle mass you have, the more calories you burn all the time.

The goal with this plan isn't just to lose total weight. The goal is to lose your body fat stores while increasing muscle mass and strength. So even though the number on the scale might stay the same or not go down as fast, you will still start to see the extra inches vanish from your waistline, and you will have the leaner, harder body you're looking for. You will have more energy and feel stronger. Most importantly, you will be healthier. With increased muscle strength, you can have a better quality of life and may even live longer.

You'll feel good, and that will make every part of your life sweeter.

Small Is Big

Your habits can be incredibly powerful. People don't realize what an enormous difference healthy decisions—or unhealthy decisions—can make in their lives, long term.

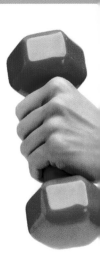

 # Think About It.

Choices might look small when you're making them on a day-to-day basis. But before you know it, a few months go by. Then a year. Then a few years. Soon, boom—twenty years have gone by, and you can really see the results of all those "insignificant" things you did in the past.

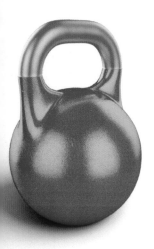

Years ago, my friend Lisa asked me to start lifting weights with her. I wasn't jumping up and down dying to lift weights, but I knew it was good for me, and I liked the idea of socializing with her. So we started hitting the gym. Lisa was consistent, so I was fairly consistent. Once a week, we lifted weights for thirty-five minutes. I thought, Thirty-five minutes, one time a week? There's no way this is making a difference.

Then a year later, I went on a ski trip with my family. I was expecting to be ambushed by aches and pains after that first day on the slopes the way I usually was after not skiing for a few years. I wasn't sore at all. I didn't get sore the next day, either. Or the day after that.

Those thirty-five minutes of weight training once a week, about 75 percent of the time, had made a real difference after all.

Habits Are a Two-Sided Coin

They can work for you, or they can work against you. And food is the same way. It can be your medicine, or it can be your poison. It can cause big inflammatory problems over time that result in excessive body fat and chronic disease, or it can keep you healthy for years at the cellular level.

Every small act you make is a choice. And optimal health starts with building healthy habits, one small action at a time. Small actions over time make big impacts on your quality of life!

The Science of Great Health

"Healthy" is Evolving

Our understanding of what it means to be healthy is evolving. Science is showing us new possibilities for health that we never considered before.

In 2011, the New England Journal of Medicine published a detailed analysis of several factors affecting the body weight of 120,877 people. Researchers followed participants for twelve to twenty years and had the individuals complete detailed questionnaires about their health habits and food intake along the way.

What they discovered was that seemingly insignificant habits in eating and exercise resulted in large changes in body weight over the years. The average participant gained almost one pound every year over the twenty years, while some lost weight during the same time.

The types of foods they ate made the biggest difference. The researchers found that the number of calories eaten didn't seem to matter as much as the kinds of calories that were consumed. Fruits, vegetables, and whole grains were common among participants who lost weight and maintained healthy weight levels. Interestingly, those who ate yogurt lost the most weight: an average of 0.82 pounds every four years, which the researchers attributed to the yogurt's healthy bacteria. Those who ate nuts and nut butters were close behind, highlighting the fact that certain high-calorie foods can actually promote weight loss.

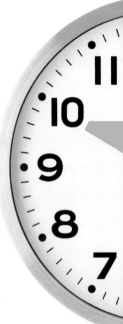

Exercise, Healthy Eating, & Sleep

Exercise and sleep also affected the weights of the participants. Participants who ate healthy and exercised gained 1.76 fewer pounds than those who didn't exercise, though active participants who ignored their diet still gained weight. Those who slept less than six hours or more than eight hours a night were usually the people who gained the most.

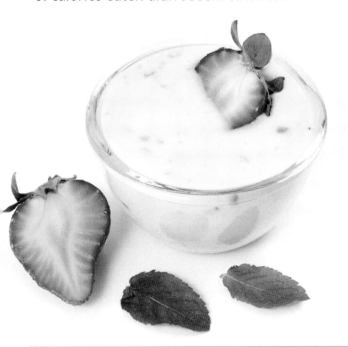

The results supported everything I was experiencing with my clients. And they were completely consistent with my 12-FIX PLAN to a leaner, healthier, happier life.

12-FIX LEAN LIFE PLAN

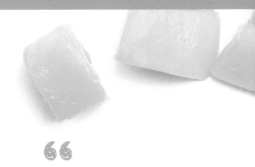

Over the years, I've identified the twelve most valuable factors involved in losing fat weight, reducing inflammation, and preventing disease. I call them the 12-FIX LEAN LIFE PLAN to boost health while juggling it all.

I've tested all twelve of these fixes on myself and on hundreds of clients. The people I work with feel better and lose inches without suffering through traditional, calorie-counting, all-or-nothing dieting routines. My own weight hasn't changed, but the people around me swear that I'm much thinner than I used to be. That's because while I haven't lost weight overall, I've lost fat weight and gained compact muscle-mass weight instead. At the age of fifty-one, I looked more toned than I had since I was in my late twenties.

My clients and I don't just look leaner. We are stronger, more positive, and more energetic than we were before we started using the twelve fixes in our day-to-day lives. We're healthier than we've been in a long time—and we feel like a million bucks.

These twelve fixes are the keys to busting fat, avoiding chronic disease, and becoming more productive. And the best part is, you don't have to follow them to the letter 100 percent of the time. Not even close. You can follow them most of the time, and you'll still make a big difference in your health as long as you do them "most of the time" consistently from now on. You never have to feel guilty, because this isn't a "diet." This is a shift in the way you think about your food and your health. It's about feeling empowered by every healthy choice you make each day, even when it seems small.

It's about feeling empowered by every healthy choice you make each day, even when it seems small.

Every healthy choice you make adds up over the years. That means that every fix you make, large or small, is going to have a positive impact on your health in the long run.

What You'll Learn

This book will take you through everything you need to know about eating deliciously nutritious foods while juggling your busy schedule.

- Which foods to track (instead of calories)
- How to time your eating for optimal results
- How small, seemingly insignificant actions you do every day or the placement of food in your environment encourages you to eat more
- Which foods to eat to burn calories and body fat
- Which foods to buy at the grocery store, restaurants, and airports
- How to prepare whole, tasty foods super fast

We will also go through two other very important aspects of health: movement and recovery. You will discover that movement can be enjoyable and fulfilling as well as efficient and effective. You'll also find out how sleep can sabotage or enhance your health. On the way, you'll find information and action plans for my twelve life-changing fixes:

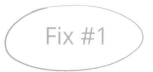

Replace sugar, refined white flour, and processed foods with whole foods.
Swap out unhealthy sweeteners such as sugar, high-fructose corn syrup, and agave nectar with healthy sweeteners such as whole fruit, raw unfiltered honey, or real maple syrup. Substitute refined flours with whole and ancient grains. Forgo commercially processed food in favor of foods in their natural form as much as possible.

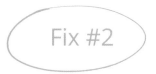

Replace less-healthy fats with healthier fats. Replace lard, butter, shortening, and margarine with monounsaturated fats such as olive oils, high-heat safflower oil, canola oil, avocado oil, and nut oils. Eat raw nuts and seeds, avocados on salads and sandwiches (instead of mayo), and sustainable fish at least twice a week to consume more omega-3 fatty acids. They are also found in walnuts, flax seeds, and chia seeds.

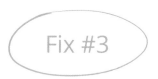

Eat a fermented food, like yogurt, every day. Try to eat or drink food containing live active bacteria, such as lower-sugar yogurt. Consistency is more important than quantity; the more regularly you eat fermented foods, the more good bacteria you'll foster in your digestive system.

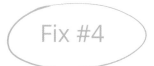

Rearrange your environment. Making some simple changes to your surroundings can trick your brain into wanting to eat less unhealthy food. Pay attention to which signals around you are encouraging you to eat the wrong types of foods in the wrong amounts. Then, you can make some switches to avoid the problems altogether. No fighting your willpower with this fix; just reorganize your home, work space, or drive home to avoid seeing unhealthy foods or use smaller plates, bowls, and spoons, for instance. The list of effective strategies goes on and on.

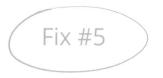

Make fruits and vegetables 50 percent of your meals and snacks. Remember that beans, lentils, dried peas, and starchy vegetables such as peas count as vegetables (except French fries and other fried potatoes). Fruits and vegetables contain powerful phytonutrients that are extremely beneficial to our health. This one fix alone can make a positive impact on your body weight and lowers disease risk too.

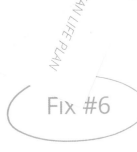

Fix #6

Eat between three and six servings of whole grains per day. A serving of grain, such as brown and black rice, farro, barley, oats, quinoa, sorghum, or whole-grain pasta, is typically half a cup or one slice of whole-grain bread. Put the emphasis on ancient grains as often as possible. Consuming enough whole grains is especially important to support activity, thinking, and digestive health. More servings may be needed on days filled with intense exercise.

Fix #7

Front-load your eating. Eat to fuel your body during the day, when you're concentrating and moving. This keeps you full and energetic all day long. Eat breakfast like a healthy king, lunch like a prince, and dinner like a pauper. Avoid eating in the evening after dinner before bed to give your body a head start on burning fat during the night.

Fix #8

Chew small bites of food slowly and completely, eat only when you're hungry, and stop eating just before you get full. Take small bites of food and chew slowly until nothing solid is left before you swallow. The more you chew, the more nutrients you absorb, calories you burn, and food you digest. Instead of eating just because it's "time" to eat, eat only when you're truly hungry and stop eating just as you become satisfied rather than being uncomfortable.

Fix #9

Drink water throughout the day and evening. Drinking water frequently and consistently ensures that the fat cells are swollen with water to keep them burning energy to their full capacity. Keep a glass or bottle of water within arm's reach at all times. If it's there, you're more likely to drink it!

Fix #10

Eat a total of 75 to 150 grams of protein spread out evenly through the day, with at least 30 grams of protein for breakfast. Protein spread throughout the day keeps you full, improves your brainpower, and helps increase muscle mass. The high-protein boost eaten (not drunk) in the morning even helps to reduce cravings for unhealthy foods in the late afternoon and evening, when willpower is weakest. Multiply your body weight in pounds by 0.6 to determine about how much protein you need to eat spread through the day.

Fix #11

Move more. Whatever movement you currently are doing, add a little more. Our amazing bodies are constantly learning and adapting. Moving more can mean more time, more frequently, more intensely, or even more variety and, thus, more fun! The more you move, the better. Each movement adds up to create optimal health.

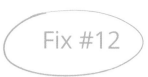

Fix #12

Sleep seven to eight hours every night. Set a time to go to bed and stick to it. If you're not tired, read a book instead of watching TV to relax. If you get enough sleep, you'll be more productive the next day. Inadequate sleep encourages higher levels of hunger hormones and decreases fat-burning and muscle-building activity during sleep. In other words, the better you manage your sleep, the better you'll be able to manage your weight.

Think About It.

These twelve fixes can transform your health and your life. Remember, this isn't a diet. You don't need to go overboard, but take these fixes seriously. Even if they seem small, over time they can make a big impact on your appearance and your health.

Take Body Measurements

Start by taking your waist measurement, and remeasure exactly the same way every month. Access a body composition test to find out your body fat and lean tissue body percentage if available. Then retest every three months.

However, if you don't have access to this test, no worries! Body measurements will suffice and are still a better indicator of your progress than the number on the scale.

Take advantage of the LEAN BODY, SMART LIFE app to provide guidance. This app offers suggestions for the fixes most advantageous to you and your struggles.

Focus Fix

Choose one of these recommended fixes to focus on each week for twelve weeks to jumpstart your

12-FIX LEAN LIFE PLAN. Once you begin a "focus fix," you should continue to follow and track it as you add new fixes each week. After twelve weeks, you should still continue to work on all twelve fixes, but concentrate on one fix a month until all twelve fixes become an integral part of your life.

Track these fixes throughout the day. Every time you make a healthy choice, you can use the LEAN BODY, SMART LIFE app to track it. Focus on your good choices, not your bad ones! Build new habits around the fixes, even if you don't follow them perfectly. Feel good about the positive changes you make, no matter how big or small they are.

Above all, remember: don't push yourself so hard that you get discouraged and give up. Cut yourself some slack, and give yourself as much positive reinforcement as possible. Perfection is not nearly as important as longevity!

Lean Body, Smart Life

The 12-FIX LEAN LIFE PLAN is based on the latest science. We know so much more about nutrition and health today than we did thirty years ago, or even five years ago. We know that it's not so much about the total calories you eat; it's more about the types of calories you choose to take in. It's less about the total body weight and more about how much of that weight is from fat and muscle.

It's Not About Being Perfect

It's about making positive changes to your health most of the time over the long term.

This plan involves eating, not starving. In fact, it's a lot of food. Almost all of my clients say that they eat more food while they are losing weight. Even better, the food tastes great, so you don't feel bad about saying no to processed foods most of the time. It's all about having tasty replacements available!

At the end of each chapter, you'll find some of my favorite recipes for healthy eating. My plan works with any diet restrictions you may already be following. It doesn't matter if you are vegetarian, vegan, nondairy, non-egg, soy-free, or gluten-free. You can weave these twelve fixes into your lifestyle for real and lasting results.

Lean Body, Smart Life isn't just a book you read. It's an action plan packed full of ways to make it easy for you to eat, move, and sleep smarter while juggling the craziness of the day. The tools in this book can empower you to transform your body shape, your health, your productivity, and your life, one easy fix at a time. Your lean body will lead to a smarter life - physically, mentally, and, even financially.

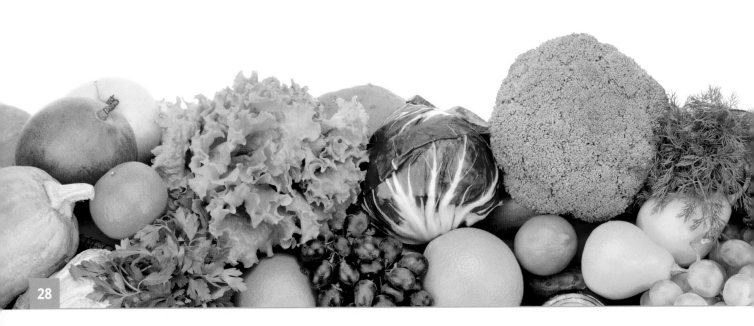

Chapter 2: Know Your Food

Visit FoodsWithJudes.com/book-content for recipes, articles and videos.

Cereal for Dessert

When my kids were in elementary school, they begged me for sweet cereal.

"Please, Mom?" they said whenever we walked through the cereal aisle at the grocery store. "We never get to have it! All my friends eat cereal every day."

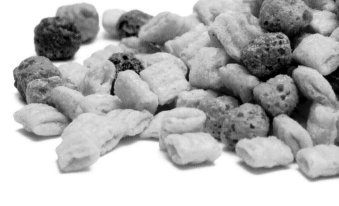

I didn't want to feed them sugar for breakfast, but I didn't want to deny the cereal altogether, either. I knew that if I never let them have it at all, they'd put it on a pedestal. Psychologically, they'd want it even more just because they couldn't have it. So I made a rule. "Yes, you can have cereal sometimes," I said, "but you can only eat it for dessert."

That was good enough for them. Once or twice a year, when their requests were extra loud, I'd let them put a few bright-colored boxes into the shopping cart. When we got home, they would write their names on their boxes in Sharpie ink – just to make sure that no one else would eat their cereal.

They would enjoy those sugary cereals at first. But they could eat them only for dessert, and most of the time we had better whole foods in the house. The processed cereals couldn't compete. After a while, they would stop eating them. A few months later, I would quietly toss out the boxes. Nobody noticed or cared.

All the while, I kept on feeding them healthy, whole foods.

Once my kids became teenagers, they didn't want sweet cereals anymore. "Mom," my youngest admitted when she was fourteen, "I feel awful when I eat sugary foods in the morning."

They all came to that realization on their own. And I knew that when they eventually went out into the world to build their lives, they were still going to make at least some healthy choices. Not because I told them to, but because they themselves learned to appreciate the value of whole, healthy foods.

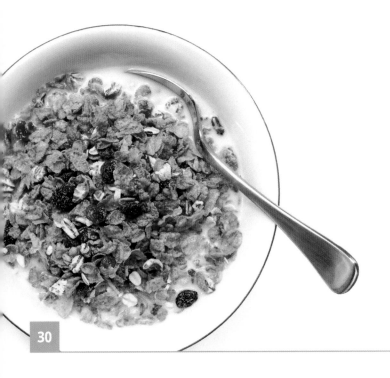

Whole Food, Super Strength

Foods in their whole form, without processing, are good for you, but you might not realize just how good they are.

Whole foods, packaged by Mother Nature, do more than just make you feel great. They also help you lose fat weight and prevent a host of health problems. For example, fruits and vegetables contain super concentrated phytonutrients that deliver a major boost to your immune system. When you eat lots of them, not only do you lose fat and reduce inflammation, you think and feel better, fight off sickness, lower your blood pressure, and reduce your risk of diseases such as cancer, diabetes, and heart disease.

> 66
>
> ...fruits and vegetables contain super-concentrated phytonutrients that deliver a major boost to your immune system.
>
> 99

Weight gain, packaged food, and inflammation are all linked. Many of the foods Americans love to eat—highly processed ones made with refined flours and sugars—are wreaking havoc in our bodies by encouraging fat cells to store those calories rather than using them for energy. This leads to more body fat and causes ongoing inflammation inside your body.

Even if you manage to keep your weight down while eating these foods, your body is still left with chronic inflammation and poor gut health. Both will make you less energetic, less able to concentrate, and eventually lead to illness of some kind down the road. Populations that adopt an American diet high in processed foods have more disease within a few years.

Your immune system can only fight off so much at once. Not only do processed foods deprive your body of valuable nutrients that help fight toxins; they add more problems for your body. All of this takes a significant toll on your immune system.

Tens of Thousands of Nutrients

Whole foods are the answer to that problem. Whole foods in their natural form are packed with tens of thousands of nutrients that work together in powerful ways, which we don't fully understand, to reduce inflammation, lower your risk of disease, and help you keep fat weight down.

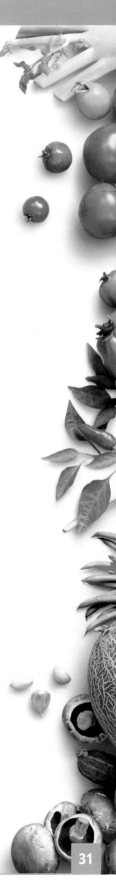

Pills can't compete with Mother Nature. Studies comparing the effectiveness of vitamins and minerals taken in supplement form versus in their natural state have shown that the supplements aren't nearly as powerful as nutrient-dense whole foods. Because all the nutrients work together in ways we don't understand, individual nutrients don't have the same impact on their own.

Did You Know?

In 1994, research established that eating deep-orange fruits and vegetables high in carotenes, such as carrots, had the power to fight cancer, especially lung cancer. Researchers assumed that the beta-carotene in supplement form could reduce the risk of cancer but were surprised to discover that beta-carotene supplements not only were useless against cancer, but actually increased the risk of cancer for people who smoked. Only natural carotene consumed from whole foods proved to be a powerful ally against the disease.

How the different nutrients in whole foods work together is still a mystery. But we do know that the structures found in nature make us healthier. More than twenty-five thousand phytonutrients are found in whole foods from plants. One apple, for instance, contains more than ten thousand nutrients laboring together to increase the ability of the apple calories to be used for energy rather than stored in fat cells. In ways researchers are just beginning to understand, all those thousands of nutrients also help decrease chronic inflammation, insulin resistance, and chronic disease.

Whole Foods in Natural Form

When you eat whole foods in their natural form, you raise your defenses against heart disease, strokes, high blood pressure, cancer, type 2 diabetes, gastrointestinal diseases, macular degeneration, and many others. Furthermore, you feel better. Your energy levels rise and your focus increases.

You can find whole foods in natural form in every branch of the food kingdom, from sugars to grains to fats to proteins. Your options for healthy eating are abundant.

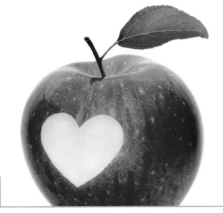

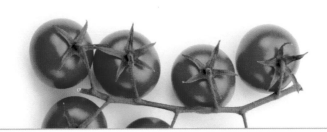

Sweet and Healthy

America Has a Sweet Tooth

We all know that we eat too much sugar and high-fructose corn syrup. We keep eating it anyway because we have become accustomed—even addicted—to the taste of processed sweets. Some studies have even reported that rats had a stronger response to sugar than they did to cocaine.

Sugar has a rap sheet a mile long. It's empty of nutrients and it's a concentrated source of calories that rush into our bloodstream too fast, inviting a flux of insulin to handle the sugar rush. That insulin surge promotes fat cells to be set in fat-making gear instead of burning mode, trapping the calories to make fat. The body responds with hunger and cravings, especially for processed carbs, because those trapped calories aren't available for energy. This cycle repeats, leading to obesity and inflammation as well as the many health problems that go along with them, including type 2 diabetes and heart disease.

The research overwhelmingly indicates that when we cut back on sugar and refined flour, many of those ill effects disappear.

We need to make a shift from processed, refined sugars to sweeteners found in their whole, natural-food forms.

Even our brains benefit from this lower-sugar shift. While our brains need carbohydrates to think, stay focused, and keep our attention from drifting, it's critical that the sugar be broken down by the body from whole foods rather than from concentrated sources of processed sugar. Without the thousands of nutrients in whole food, sugar is absorbed too quickly, leading to a burst of energy followed by a slump. Sugar eaten in whole foods, however, results in a more consistent, longer-lasting energy source for the brain to think clearly, longer.

The healthiest sweeteners for us are whole-food sweeteners that deliver vitamins, minerals, phytonutrients, and fiber along with their sweet taste. We want to eat whole foods in natural form, and sweeteners are no exception. Fruit, raw unfiltered honey, real maple syrup, and dark chocolate or cocoa all fit the bill for natural sweeteners that help negate the bad effects of the natural sugar they contain.

Whole Fruit Sauce or Syrup

Commercial pancake syrup is a processed food that many people have a hard time letting go. Luckily, whole fruit makes a perfect substitute. Throw some fresh or frozen fruit into a saucepan with a little bit of juice and cook it down while you're making your pancakes. Add a little raw honey or real maple syrup if the fruit needs sweetening. In ten minutes, you have soft syrup with chunks of soft fruit. I usually add a tablespoon of chia seeds to the fruit mixture to help it thicken while adding nutrition.

The high number of antioxidants in the chia seeds helps the leftover fruit syrup last longer in the refrigerator too. I often add this leftover fruit mixture to my plain Greek yogurt. Try natural, unsweetened applesauce to add sweetness and moisture to baked goods.

"Dessert" Dates

Dates are packed with vitamins and minerals, including B6, A, K, niacin, riboflavin, folate, potassium, magnesium, manganese, iron, zinc, and calcium. Each date you eat contains almost two grams of fiber, which slows down the absorption of sugar into the bloodstream. Dates are also rich in protein: they contain five times more protein than any other fruit. They are an excellent source of antioxidants, and they contain twenty-three amino acids. Dates are the most nutritious sweetener we have, and they are easiest to include when you are already using a high-powered blender for your recipe. The more you can replace sugar with whole foods such as naturally sweet dates, the better it will be for your health.

Read More About Dates

Raw Honey

Honey is also loaded with vitamins, minerals, phytonutrients, and living enzymes with antiviral and antibacterial properties—but it has to be raw. These valuable nutrients are destroyed during the heating and pasteurization process in commercially processed honey, which causes it to rush into the bloodstream as sugar does.

The glycemic index (GI) is a ranking of carbohydrates in foods according to how they affect blood sugar levels. Carbohydrates with a GI value of 55 or less out of 100 are more slowly digested, absorbed, and metabolized, thus causing a lower and slower rise in blood sugar and, therefore, insulin levels. Lower insulin levels keep fat cells in burn mode rather than store and grow mode.

In fact, processed sugar and honey have similar high glycemic index ratings, around 70 to 90. By contrast, raw honey has a glycemic index rating of about 30 to 40 according to the Glycemic Index Database. Not only does raw honey promote a more stable blood sugar level, but because it's sweeter than other sugars, you can use about 25 percent less of it when sweetening your foods and drinks.

Read More About The Benefits of Raw Honey

Did You Know?

No honey for babies. Never give any kind of honey to a child under one year of age. An infant's immune system can't deactivate the botulinum spores found in honey. These spores may grow in the digestive tract and produce toxins, which will make the infant sick.

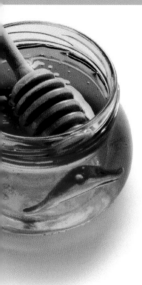

Real Maple Syrup

Real maple syrup tapped from trees, not the commercial pancake syrups made from high-fructose corn syrup, is a healthy, natural sweetener as well. While the body breaks down the sugar a little faster than it does raw honey, it's still slower than table sugar or processed honey (glycemic index rating of about 50). It may not provide as many phytonutrients or as much fiber as crushed fruit does, but it's easy to use and adds a delicious flavor.

Dark Chocolate and Cocoa

Unsweetened cooking cocoa can be eaten frequently. I even add cocoa to my chili. Homemade desserts made with cocoa are better for you if you use a more nutritious sweetener and fat source. Dark chocolate contains not only cocoa but also cocoa butter and sugar, so it needs to be limited to a small amount. However, that small amount of dark chocolate eaten regularly is a positive habit. Dark chocolate and cocoa are full of antioxidants (even more than kale and spinach) and may also have anticancer properties.

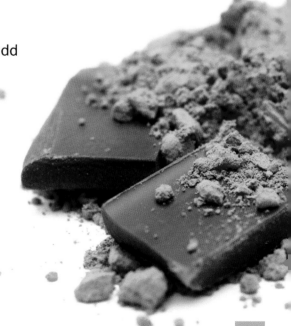

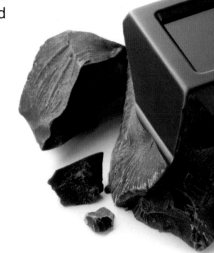

They contain flavonoids, which boost heart health by reducing bad cholesterol levels and keep your arteries flexible to increase blood flow and lower blood pressure.

The less processed your dark chocolate is, the better. Avoid chocolate where sugar is listed as the first ingredient. Aim for a 70 percent cocoa content or higher in your dark chocolate to get the greatest amount of disease-fighting flavonoids out of it. And remember not to overdo it. Even though it has many nutritious properties, dark chocolate is also cocoa butter. Stick with just a square or two a day.

Read More About Dark Chocolate and Cocoa

 # Think About It.

Some sweeteners start out healthy in nature, but by the time you buy them, they have been highly processed. Agave nectar is presented as a healthy, natural sweetener because it doesn't stimulate insulin the way glucose does. But agave nectar is 90 percent fructose. That's even more fructose than high-fructose corn syrup, which has a fructose content of 55 percent. Fructose in processed foods is absorbed quickly without Mother Nature's packaging and ends up promoting dangerous belly fat.

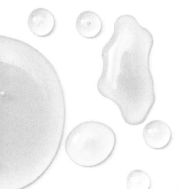

Artificial Sweeteners

Although artificial sweeteners have essentially no calories, they do affect the body. Our sweetness taste receptors perceive them to be hundreds to thousands of times sweeter than sugar. Those who consume these synthetic chemicals may find naturally sweet food less appealing. Artificial sweeteners may also increase insulin, causing calories to be shifted to fat cells rather than burned for energy.

If you have to use an artificial sweetener, I recommend monk fruit sweetener, and even then, it's almost always better to eat fruit in its whole form. The monk fruit is an ancient Chinese fruit two hundred to three hundred times sweeter than sugar. However, by the time it reaches the grocery store shelf, it has still been refined and processed. Too bad we can't just buy the fruit!

Whole and Ancient Grains

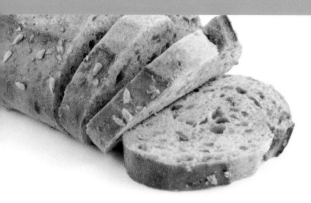

Fruits and vegetables aren't the only things packed full of nutrients. Whole grains are too—especially when they're ancient grains.

Carbohydrates have gotten a bad reputation, and processed grains deserve it. Besides being absorbed very quickly into the bloodstream and putting your body in fat-making gear, refined flour and white rice are stripped of their bran and germ. The bran and germ are loaded with vitamins, minerals, fiber, and thousands of disease-fighting phytonutrients. Whole grains take longer than processed grains to break down. That means that the bloodstream absorbs them more slowly, resulting in more stable blood sugars for better hunger control, long-lasting energy, and more constant fuel for your brain to function at its peak for longer. It's not surprising that whole grains have been shown to reduce the risk of heart disease, type 2 diabetes, obesity, and even some forms of cancer.

All Whole Grains Are Good in Moderation

Some whole grains pack an extra punch. Ancient grains are grains that have been around for millennia. While corn, rice, and modern wheat have been bred selectively over time, ancient grains still have a composition similar to what they had thousands of years ago, which can be beneficial to your body.

Ancient grains include quinoa, sorghum, farro, amaranth, einkorn, millet, spelt, teff, freekeh, and Kamut. If you're looking for a good place to start experimenting, sorghum is gluten-free and one of my favorites. It has a nice, neutral flavor like that of rice.

Farro, another favorite, is bigger in size than some other ancient grains so that it feels more satisfying to chew. The pearled version only takes only fifteen minutes to cook and still contains 5 grams of fiber and 7 grams of protein in just over a half a cup cooked. As a bonus, the wheat-based ancient grains, like farro, tend to be lower in gluten than their modern-day counterparts.

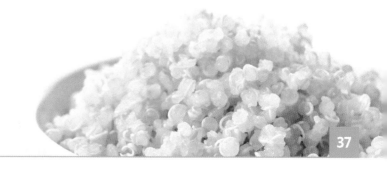

Gluten-Free Grains

Gluten has become a much bigger problem for many people in recent years. Food companies add vital wheat gluten to bread, including whole-grain varieties, for the airy fluff needed to compensate for shortcut commercial mixing that takes three hours to produce a loaf of bread instead of days like it used to. It doesn't stop there; gluten is added to pastas, snacks, cereals, and crackers, and as a thickener in hundreds of foods to increase shelf life and act as a binder. The excessive amounts of high-gluten processed foods appear to be negatively affecting our health.

Just changing foods to their whole form and concentrating on ancient grains is enough for many to improve their health. Others may need to avoid gluten in their diets by replacing processed foods with gluten-free whole grains to feel better. Those with celiac disease need to completely eliminate gluten from what they eat. Beware: gluten-free processed food is still processed food, so don't be lulled into the notion that it's good for you! Grains close to their whole-food form, rather than processed food, are the healthiest way to eat within almost any diet restriction.

66

Grains close to their whole-food form, rather than processed food, are the healthiest way to eat within almost any diet restriction.

99

Quinoa, brown and black rice, and sorghum are delicious examples of gluten-free whole grain for those needing to eliminate gluten. You have plenty of great-tasting and easy-to-fix whole grains at your disposal.

Gluten-free whole grains (or in some cases seeds or grasses) that act like grains include the following:

- Quinoa

- Sorghum

- Whole-grain corn

- Oats (must be labeled gluten-free)

- Popcorn

- Brown rice

- Wild rice

- Black rice

- Amaranth

- Buckwheat

- Millet

- Teff

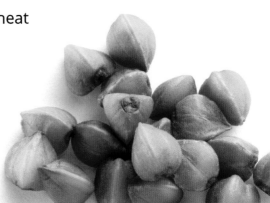

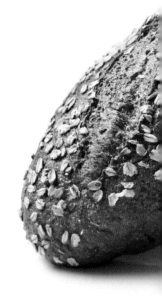

Low-FODMAP Diet

Many people who feel better on a gluten-free diet don't realize that the carbohydrates in the wheat may be causing their intestinal distress, rather than an issue with eating gluten. Certain carbohydrates, but not just the carbs in wheat, are harder to absorb into your body. For some people, this can cause digestive problems.

These particular carbohydrates are referred to by the acronym FODMAP. These carbohydrates are found in some foods and are not always tolerated in people with Irritable Bowel Syndrome (IBS) or other gut issues. However, these carbs (like certain types of fruits, wheat, dairy, and legumes to name a few) are healthy, well-tolerated foods for most people.

The low-FODMAP diet eliminates these types of carbohydrates for a short time and then adds them back in one at a time. This can help identify the types of specific carbohydrates that might cause intestinal problems for that individual. These groups of carbohydrates tend to provide important nourishment for your health-promoting gut bacteria. Therefore, it's critical to find out which groups are not a problem for you, so that they can be added back into your diet. The low-FODMAP diet is medically based, and is used and researched all over the world for those with IBS and other intestinal issues. It requires individual guidance by a registered dietitian nutritionist.

If you know which diet you truly need to be on, you can benefit from more options with less intestinal discomfort. For instance, If you are on a low-FODMAP diet, you can usually eat some types of sourdough bread. You can improve your digestive symptoms, but can still allow yourself a variety of options that can improve your health.

Recent diets have been popping up that may be an oblivious extension of the low-FODMAP diet. These fad diets eliminate whole food groups unnecessarily. Eliminating sugar is a good thing, but eliminating all dairy, grains (including whole ancient grains), and legumes is usually unnecessary and less healthy. In fact, the low-FODMAP diet still allows yogurt, kefir, hard cheeses even though most dairy products are excluded for a trial time. Those important details get lost in the oversimplification of the low-FODMAP diet.

> If you want to eliminate a whole category of food, exclude sugar, refined grains (like white flour), and processed food!

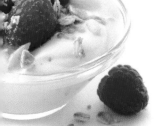

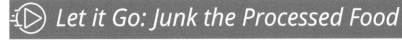 *Let it Go: Junk the Processed Food*

FIX #1

Replace Sugar, Refined White Flour, and Processed Foods with Whole Foods

If you're ready to lose weight, reduce inflammation, and feel and think better, the first step is simple: eat less sugar and food made with white flour. When you eat less, you'll want less. Processed foods encourage us to crave sugar and refined carbs. Because my kids weren't used to eating sweet cereal and I only let them have it occasionally for dessert, they didn't establish a taste for it. The more you avoid sugar and processed food, the less you'll want it over time.

Processed food is filled with sugar and high-fructose corn syrup—even when it's not sweet. Prepared salad dressings, boxed mixes, processed syrup, cookies, bread, you name it: if it's not prepared by you, it probably has sugar or high-fructose corn syrup in it.

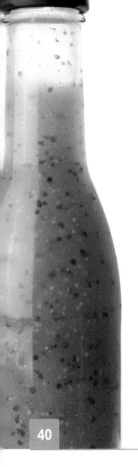

Replace refined, processed sugar and high-fructose corn syrup with natural sweeteners such as whole fresh fruit, raw unfiltered honey, or real maple syrup. Replace white flour with whole-grain flour and swear off white bread and buns as much as possible! And of course, make an effort to eat all of your food in whole form, such as whole-grain bread or plain yogurt mixed with a little real maple syrup and topped with fruit and nuts.

 ## Think About It

This one fix alone can be a game changer. My clients drop several inches from their waistlines by cutting back on sugar, white bread, white rice, and pasta alone. Even when they're not super strict about it, they still lose weight over the course of several months. Remember, it's never all or nothing. If you eat a slice of white bread at a restaurant one day, don't use the slip as an excuse to go back to eating it all the time.

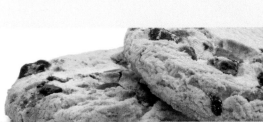

Fix #1 Action Plan:

✓ *Cut out sugar completely for two weeks to dull your cravings for sweet things. When you need to eat something sweet, eat a fruit in its whole form.*

✓ *Skip white bread altogether. Replace foods made with white flour—such as crackers and bread—with whole grains.*

✓ *Replace white rice and pasta with brown rice and whole-grain pasta. Or replace these processed foods with ancient grains such as sorghum, farro, or quinoa.*

✓ *When you need to use sugar in cooking or baking, use crushed or cooked-down fruit, raw honey, or a little real maple syrup (not processed syrup). If you're using a high-powered blender for your recipe, replace sugar with pitted dates.*

✓ *Don't live without chocolate if you want it. Just eat no more than one to two squares of it in a day, and make sure it has a 70 percent cocoa content or higher. There is no limit on cocoa, however. Add cocoa to recipes such as stew, chili, and oatmeal.*

✓ *Order brown rice instead of white rice in restaurants.*

✓ *Replace white potatoes with purple and sweet potatoes, which have a lower glycemic index rating and help with inflammation.*

Track Your Progress on The LEAN BODY, SMART LIFE App

The Facts About Fats

Let me set you straight on fats. We've spent decades conditioning everyone to think of fats as a bad thing and to follow low-fat diets. It turns out that we were way off. Even though fat has more than twice as many calories as carbohydrates and proteins, the type of fat makes the big difference, not the calories. Certain types of fat are actually good for you, and despite the concentrated calories, can help you lose body fat.

Unhealthy saturated fat, on the other hand, appears to increase chronic inflammation (including inflammation of the region of the brain that regulates hunger and metabolism) and the need for insulin, as well as body fat and chronic disease. If we replace unhealthy saturated fats, such as animal fat in meats and fats used in refined and processed foods, with good fats, such as canola or olive oil, we will be way ahead of the game. The saturated fats found in dairy products appear to be more of a neutral fat, not as harmful as once thought but not nearly as helpful in improving health as omega-3 fatty acids and monounsaturated fats.

Two types of fat, omega-3 fatty acids and monounsaturated fats, can actually help our bodies lower inflammation and burn calories. Even better, these healthy fats taste great and can be more satisfying than less-healthy fats, too!

Omega-3 Fatty Acids

The active forms of omega-3 fatty acids, DHA and EPA, are found almost exclusively in ocean algae and fish that have eaten algae, such as salmon and seaweed. The inactive and less effective form of omega-3 fatty acids (ALA) is found in some plant-based foods such as walnuts, flax, chia seeds, and canola oil. While ALA is still valuable, the body can utilize only about 5 percent of it.

Because omega-3 fatty acids are not made by the body, they must be obtained from food. It is essential that we eat them! Ideally, the active forms of omega-3s should come from the recommended two to three seafood meals or at least eight ounces of seafood (which can include canned salmon or tuna) each week, with omega-3 fatty acid supplements used as needed. Don't replace seafood with fish oil supplements if you can avoid it. While fish oil pills are helpful, recent research has indicated that the benefits from eating seafood exceed those of supplements. Plus, while fish oil supplements provide omega-3 fatty acids, they don't contain all of the many other hard-to-find nutrients found in seafood.

These powerful omega-3 fatty acids decrease chronic inflammation and seem to help fight inflammatory diseases such as arthritis and irritable bowel syndrome. They can also inhibit cancer and protect your heart. Omega-3s reduce deaths from heart disease, especially sudden deaths. Some omega-3s protect against abnormal heart rhythms, lower the risk of blood clots, reduce triglycerides, decrease the growth of plaque on artery walls, and reduce the risk of a stroke.

Omega-3s protect brain function. They seem to be especially important for a well-functioning central nervous system and for the transmission of signals from the eyes to the brain. The omega-3 fatty acid DHA is integral to a baby's brain development and function, as well as for the development of the retina in the eye and the vascular system. Omega-3s are critical for learning, vision, and brain function. Studies have indicated that breastfed babies with the highest omega-3 DHA levels have cognitive and IQ advantages.

Omega-3s are important for mental health too. Low omega-3 fatty acid DHA levels are associated with depression, memory loss, dementia, and visual problems. Low DHA levels during pregnancy can increase the mother's risk for postpartum depression. Inadequate maternal intake of omega-3 fatty acids may increase the risk of childhood food allergies.

For More Specifics About Omega-3s, Read Seafood News Flash

Monounsaturated Fats

Monounsaturated fatty acids, known as omega-9 fatty acids, are also "good fats." These fats decrease bad cholesterol (LDL), increase good cholesterol (HDL), lower triglycerides, blood pressure, and also help to control blood sugars. Exciting research suggests that monounsaturated fat may even help us reduce abdominal fat. Studies out of the University of Manitoba in Canada have shown that substituting monounsaturated fatty acids for the saturated fats in your diet can help you lose belly fat.

Monounsaturated fatty acids are in olive oil, refined (also known as high-heat) safflower oil, canola oil, avocados and avocado oil, peanuts and peanut oil, and tree nuts and other nut oils. These are easy to use when preparing meals and snacks.

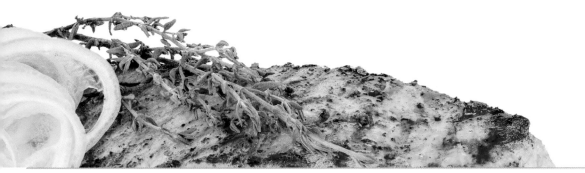

Get The Scoop on These Healthy Oils

You may be surprised at the oils that can handle heat in the kitchen!

Remember, whole foods are best. Avocados and nuts in their whole forms are an even better way to eat these. Other sources of monounsaturated fatty acids are olives, macadamia nuts, hazelnuts, pecans, almonds, cashews, Brazil nuts, pistachio nuts, pine nuts, and sesame seeds.

Olive Oil

Olive oil has plenty of well-documented health benefits. It is rich in monounsaturated fats and loaded with healthy phytonutrients. However, not all olive oils are created equal, and their many nutrients need to be protected from light and excessive heat.

Olive oil contains omega-9 fatty acids and polyphenols that lower our risk of metabolic syndrome, reduce inflammation and cell damage, and protect us from infections. The less processing the oil undergoes, the more nutrients it contains. Extra-virgin olive oil is pressed only one time without any heat, which is where it gets its beneficial reputation.

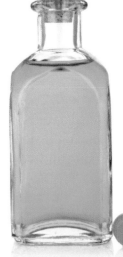

 Did You Know?

Cooking with olive oil is a different story. When extra-virgin olive oil heats up over anywhere from 300°F to 375°F (depending on the manufacturer), it breaks down chemically and loses many of its phytonutrients. You should use extra-virgin olive oil only for low-heat cooking and salad dressing. When you are cooking over moderate heat, use virgin olive oil. For higher heat, use light olive oil or just olive oil.

Keep in mind that the nutrient content of olive oils diminishes as the days, weeks, and months go by. Olive oil has a maximum shelf life of two years from the time of harvest. If the olive oil you're looking at is dated more than a year from its harvest date, don't buy it.

Learn More About Olive Oils

Butter is Not Back

Recently the phrase "Butter is Back" has been making headlines. Despite this and similar articles selling the notion that saturated fat is good for us, it's not. The major study that set off these misleading articles was a 2014 review and analysis of twenty-seven trials and forty-nine observational studies from the University of Cambridge. Several researchers in the field took issue with the deep flaws in this study. Dr. Walter Willett, Harvard's Nutrition Department chair, was alarmed by several issues. The study left out results that conflicted with its conclusions, and misrepresented some of its data. The study also neglected to consider the significant benefits of omega fats, so it missed the critical benefits of replacing saturated fats with healthier fats.

Dr. David Katz from Yale explains that this study only showed that the rate of heart disease hasn't decreased in the US, despite our small decrease in saturated fat consumption. Dr. Katz, like many other researchers, is quick to point out that it doesn't mean saturated fat isn't a problem. The real reason heart disease didn't decrease is because Americans replaced saturated fat with sugar and refined grains rather than with vegetables and whole grains.

Saturated fats aren't all the same, and they can vary in their effects on disease. Some saturated fats, like dairy fat and less-processed virgin coconut oil, appear to be less problematic. These saturated fats are more neutral than they are helpful, however. Spend your effort eating fats that improve your health and help you lose body fat.

Eating less saturated fat isn't enough. Replace butter, bacon, fatty meats, mayo, margarine, cream, and fried foods with more health-promoting fats as often as possible. Whole foods like olives, avocados, nuts, seeds, and fatty fish contain healthy polyunsaturated and monounsaturated fats. Use avocado instead of mayo or nuts instead of croutons, for instance. When you need to cook with fat, go with olive oil or another plant-based oil instead of butter or bacon fat.

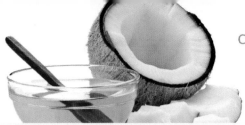

Coconut Oil

While touted as a superfood, coconut oil just doesn't stand up to the excellent benefits of both omega-3 fatty acids and monounsaturated fats. Much of coconut oil's positive health contributions are attributed to its high content of medium-chain fatty acids (MCFAs), which tend to be absorbed and metabolized more efficiently than other fats and contain six to twelve carbons. Yet the medium-chain triglycerides (MCTs) (containing twelve carbons) in coconut oil act more like typical long-chain fatty acids even though structurally they are considered medium. Long-chain fatty acids need to be broken up and packaged in lipoprotein particles that transport fat around the body.

While the traditional diets of Pacific Islanders historically included a lot of saturated fat from coconut products and the populations exhibited low incidences of cardiovascular disease, this is not sufficient to support coconut oil's superfoods status. These groups of islanders were eating grated coconut flesh, coconut cream, and coconut flour, not coconut oil. Unlike coconut oil, these coconut foods are rich in fiber, explaining in part why these groups had a lower rate of heart disease. Importantly, their traditional diets also contained plenty of fish, fruit, and vegetables, and little to no refined sugar, processed foods, or soft drinks.

Other points supporting coconut's elevated health status also have similarly strong counterpoints, but I think you get the idea. Unrefined coconut oil isn't bad for you. It appears to be a fairly neutral oil similar to the fat in dairy, but it's by no means a superfood. And it's not nearly as beneficial to your health as omega-3 fatty acids eaten in fish and monounsaturated fats eaten in nuts, seeds, olives, and avocados. I use unrefined coconut oil from time to time in some of my recipes for its taste and texture, but more often than not I use monounsaturated fats (olive oil, high-heat safflower oil, canola oil, avocados and avocado oil, peanut butter and peanut oil, and tree nut and other nut oils) for greater benefits.

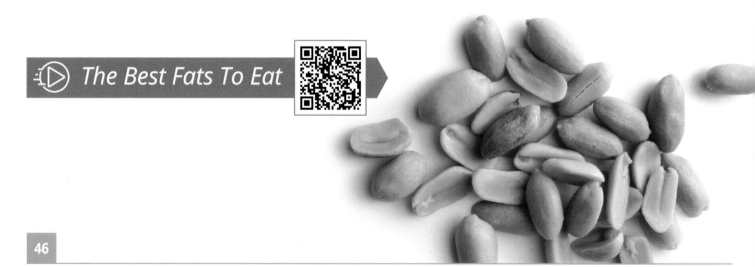

▷ *The Best Fats To Eat*

FIX #2

Replace Less-Healthy Fats with Healthier Fats

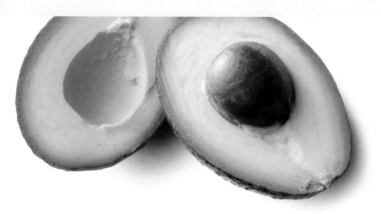

For many years, fat was considered bad for our health. However, scientific research has since shown that many kinds of fat are actually beneficial for our weight and health.

Our job is to replace less-healthy fats in our diets with healthier ones. Cut back on or get rid of meat, lard, butter, shortening, margarine, mayonnaise, cream, and sour cream. Replace them with fish, olive oil, canola oil, high-heat safflower oil, macadamia oil and other nut oils, avocado oil, and peanut oil.

Eat raw nuts and avocados frequently to increase your intake of healthy fats. Try to eat seafood, especially wild Pacific salmon, sardines, and anchovies, at least twice a week in order to consume more omega-3 fatty acids in their whole form. Flax, walnuts, chia seeds, and canola oil are also high in omega-3 fatty acids, although a less potent form that the body has to convert into the potent active DHA form.

If you can't replace all of your less-healthy fats with good ones right away, don't stress about it. Just work on gradually replacing questionable ones with healthier ones over time. Nothing in this plan is all or nothing. Every change you make will help you—even if it's small!

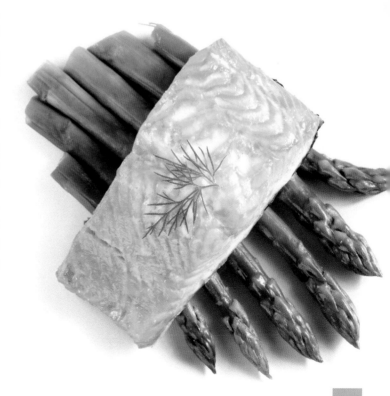

Fix #2 Action Plan:

✓ Use extra-virgin olive oil for salad dressings but higher-heat oils such as light olive oil, canola oil, avocado oil, or refined safflower oil for cooking with high heat.

✓ Replace butter in baking with canola oil, refined safflower oil, or nut butters.

✓ Replace sour cream with plain Greek yogurt.

✓ Skip store-bought salad dressings and mix one part olive oil with one part balsamic vinegar. Add salt and pepper and a little Dijon mustard. Shake vigorously for an easy dressing.

✓ Replace mayonnaise in sandwiches and other foods with avocado that is lightly salted and as slices or as a spread.

✓ Eat healthy, sustainable seafood at least twice a week. Prepare with light olive oil instead of butter.

✓ Replace butter with olive oil, refined safflower oil, canola oil, or avocado oil in cooking.

✓ Add avocado to green salads to increase your nutrient intake.

✓ Replace croutons in your salad with nuts.

✓ Eat raw nuts for a healthy snack.

Track Your Progress on The LEAN BODY, SMART LIFE App

The Power of Protein

Protein is a big power player in creating maximal health. Most of us eat enough of it to get by, but at the end of the day, we fall far short of the optimal amount of the type of protein needed to keep fat off and to maximize our movements during the day to build muscle.

When we eat enough protein, we feel less hungry and more satisfied. Around the ages of twenty-five to thirty, we start to lose muscle mass every year. Without enough protein spread out over the day to supply the necessary amino acids, we can't build valuable lean tissue to fight off that muscle loss. And those muscles burn calories for us twenty-four hours a day, seven days a week—even when we're at rest. That helps us achieve and maintain a healthy weight.

The body doesn't make all of the essential amino acids that it needs. Nine of them come from protein sources such as seafood, poultry, meat, eggs, milk and milk products, quinoa, soybeans, and amaranth. While beans, dried peas, lentils, nuts, and peanuts don't contain all nine amino acids, they are fairly high in protein and are excellent protein foods. The incomplete proteins can easily be paired with another incomplete protein such as rice or corn tortillas to guarantee intake of all the necessary amino acids. If you eat a variety of foods including vegetables and whole grains, it's easy to take in missing essential amino acids. Or simply eat a complete and healthy protein, such as yogurt or fish, along with them.

 Think About It.

Eat health-promoting protein at every meal and snack, and try to spread your protein out through the day. If your proportion of protein is out of balance, consume more of it earlier in the day, rather than in the evening as is typically done in the U.S. Also important is eating less of your protein from meat and poultry and more from seafood, plants (such as dried peas, beans, lentils, and nuts), eggs, and yogurt as recommended in the 2015–2020 USDA Dietary Guidelines for Americans that accompany MyPlate.

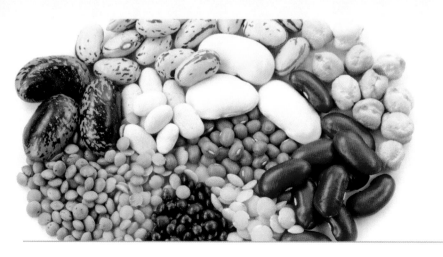
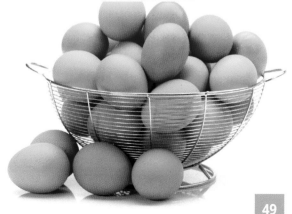

Seafood Surprise

Seafood is surprisingly proving to be the real superfood. USDA guidelines recommend eating two to three seafood meals (eight to twelve ounces) per week. The research on seafood's health benefits are very strong and the mercury issues associated with seafood are now clearer and easier to maneuver (see chapter 7).

Mercury toxicity is not an issue in most varieties of seafood, contrary to what was once suspected. Eating fish doesn't cause mercury toxicity; it actually prevents it! The selenium found in most seafood neutralizes the mercury and other toxins, and you often end up with a surplus of selenium reserves for more health benefits.

Seafood has other valuable nutrients besides quality protein and selenium. Seafood and sea vegetables (such as seaweed) are the only source of active omega-3 fatty acids (DHA and EPA). These omega-3s along with choline, vitamin D, and iodine are nutrients found in seafood that most people are not eating enough and that are difficult to find in other foods. Fish oils do supplement the active omega-3s, but don't replace all the other valuable nutrients found in fish.

Pregnant women and young children are especially in need of these valuable nutrients but are often unaware of seafood's terrific health benefits. For everyone, eating sustainable marine life is more important to your health than you can imagine!

Dairy Protein

Whey protein, found in milk, is easily absorbed and retained by the body. It's also the richest source of leucine—an amino acid that triggers muscle building. Cottage cheese has the most leucine of any dairy food with about 28 grams of protein per cup. Greek and Icelandic yogurts are also concentrated source of protein with more than double the amount of protein found in traditional yogurt.

As you increase your protein intake, it is important to eat calcium-packed foods (such as yogurt) when possible to protect your bones. Eating high protein without enough calcium (at least 600 mg/day) can lead to bone loss. But the combination of protein and calcium foods strengthens the skeleton, decreasing both osteopenia and osteoporosis later in life.

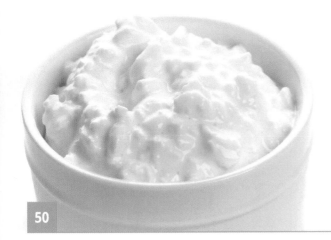

Visit Seafood News Flash for Details

Yogurt Power

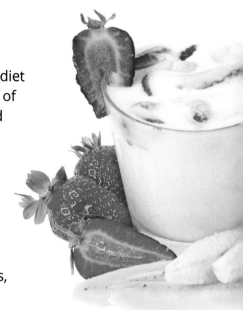

Yogurt's power to improve your health may be worth including in your diet even if you don't tolerate dairy foods. Yogurt is an efficient, easy way of taking in enough muscle-enhancing protein during the day. Other needed nutrients, such as calcium, potassium, phosphorous, vitamin D, and B12, come along for the ride. Dairy is linked to improved bone health in children and adolescents and a reduced risk of cardiovascular disease and type 2 diabetes as well as lower blood pressure in adults. Yogurt eaters in particular have been found to have lower circulating triglycerides, glucose levels, blood pressure, and insulin resistance than non-yogurt consumers. Don't forget the Harvard study mentioned in Chapter 1 that found yogurt to have the greatest impact for weight loss, with 120,877 US women and men followed over twenty years.

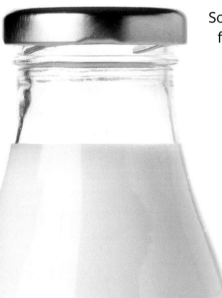

Some are opposed to dairy, but the truth is that the powerful probiotics in fermented dairy, such as yogurt and kefir, may counter and even surpass the perceived health negatives of milk products. Of course, some people are allergic to the protein in milk and shouldn't add it back to their diet. However, for those who are lactose intolerant or who have sensitivity to dairy, fermented dairy may be a viable option and well worth a try. Yogurt is low in lactose because the good bacteria in it break the lactose down during fermentation. Kefir is even better: the bacteria in it are so strong that it's actually 99 percent lactose-free.

Don't completely give up on dairy until you've given grass-fed dairy a chance. The feed given to the cows to eat may be part of the problems leading to some dairy intolerance. If you're not allergic to milk, don't miss out on these healthful ways to take in needed nutrient-loaded protein with gut-restoring probiotics in whole-food form to boost your health.

 One Food That Will Help Your Whole Body

FIX #3

Eat a Fermented Food, Like Yogurt, Every Day

We're conditioned to fear germs, yet there are as many bacteria as there are human cells in our bodies, and certain species of bacteria help us to digest our food, stay healthy and keep weight off. Our digestive tract needs to house plenty of these helpful bacteria to at least balance out the harmful ones. Primarily the food we eat determines our gut microbiota profile or microbiome. We need to replenish the good bacteria in our gut regularly by eating foods with helpful microbes—fermented foods.

Fermentation is the process where bacteria feed on the sugars in foods and release a lot of lactic acid, which helps our bodies to digest, absorb, and assimilate nutrients. Fermented foods containing live microbes help keep beneficial bacteria in good supply, to develop and maintain a healthy GI tract and boost our immune systems. Gut bacteria even create nutrients, including biotin and vitamins B12 and vitamin K.

These beneficial bacteria lower intestinal inflammation and aid digestion, as well as play a role in keeping our weight under control. Several studies have reported that the microbial populations in the gut are different between lean and heavy people, and that when heavy people lose weight, their microorganisms become similar to those of lean people. In fact, when the gut bacteria of pairs of twins, where one was lean and one was obese, were transplanted into mice, the mice that got the lean twins' bacteria remained lean, while the mice that got the obese twins' bacteria became fatter, even though they ate the same amount.

The impact on your brain function is becoming more apparent. Research is beginning to indicate that our gut microbe content affects our mental responses. Live microbes in yogurt can lead to significant improvements in depression, anger, and anxiety. Findings from UCLA research have indicated that bacteria in yogurt may actually change the way our brains respond to our environments, and can even improve brain function.

Yogurt is full of good bacteria, so add it to your diet on a daily basis when possible. Quality cheese is often created, in part, by adding live bacteria cultures, fermenting the milk's natural sugars into anti-inflammatory lactic acid. Romano (Pecorino Romano), Gouda, some cheddars, Parmesan cheese (Parmigiano-Reggiano), and even cottage cheese are made using this method. Many of these cheeses still contain some live bacteria. Cottage cheese doesn't usually contain live strains of microbes once pasteurized but may still be a benefit to your health just from being made with bacteria.

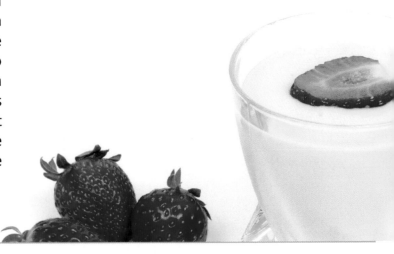

Both yogurt and kefir can be completely dairy-free when fermented with nondairy milks such as soy, almond, rice, or coconut milk. Most of these nondairy yogurts won't provide nearly as much protein or calcium, but they are fermented foods that can be helpful to our health.

Other nondairy foods, such as unpasteurized sauerkraut, olives, Korean kimchi, soy sauce, pickles (not made with vinegar but authentic fermented pickles), pickled vegetables, olives, and soybean products (tempeh, miso, and natto) are fermented. However, they may not contain nearly the gut-restoring probiotic strength that yogurt and kefir do.

The live bacteria are sensitive to heat and time, so many of these foods are void of live cultures when you buy them at the store. Look for fresh sauerkraut and olives at your deli. Kimchi is fermented and pickled cabbage mixed with other ingredients. Fermented vegetables in jars have been heat-treated, so the live cultures have been destroyed. Fresh kimchi can often be found at Asian markets and restaurants. You can also buy unpasteurized miso paste in the refrigerated section of a grocery store.

When it comes to fermented foods, how often you eat them is more important than how many of them you eat. Eating fermented foods regularly replenishes the bacteria in our digestive systems and keeps us healthy. Be consistent, and try to eat at least one fermented food every day.

Learn More About Fermented Foods

Prebiotics

While probiotic foods contain live bacteria, prebiotic foods are fiber parts of plants that we can't digest, so they become food for the good bacteria already living in our digestive systems. Studies report that eating more prebiotics positively affects your health by supporting your microbiota. By feeding good bacteria, prebiotic foods help reduce your appetite, lower your body fat, improve your glucose tolerance, and help your mood.

Include a variety of prebiotics in your diet to provide food for different strains of healthy bacteria. Prebiotics are found in certain fruits, vegetables, and whole grains. These can include whole wheat, whole barley, oatmeal, avocados, asparagus, Jerusalem artichokes, less ripe bananas, soybeans, legumes, jicama, chicory root, dandelion greens, okra, radishes, onions, garlic, leeks, chives, scallions. Raw honey, pure maple syrup, and apple cider vinegar also help feed disease-fighting gut bacteria.

Each type of prebiotic promotes the growth of different kinds of helpful bacteria, so a diet that has a variety of fiber sources supports microbiome diversity. Whole plant foods contain polyphenols. These phytochemicals are nutrients in fruits and vegetables that can slow the growth of toxic bacteria. This allows good bacteria to grow and helps prevent harmful microbes from taking over. Another reason to eat more produce!

Fix #3 Action Plan:

√ *Eat fermented foods containing live cultures regularly to replenish your gut bacteria.*

√ *Add low-sugar varieties of Greek and Icelandic yogurt and kefir to your diet daily.*

√ *Add your own sweetener to plain yogurt, such as pureed fruit, raw honey, or real maple syrup.*

√ *Try making your own yogurt. It's easy, inexpensive, and delicious.*

√ *Eat lots of fruits, vegetables, and whole grains to slow down bad bacteria growth and provide food for good bacteria.*

√ *Include a variety of prebiotics foods in your diet on a regular basis.*

√ *Mix a cup of hot water with a tablespoon of organic raw apple cider vinegar and a little raw local honey or maple syrup for a prebiotic boost. Add a squeeze of fresh lemon juice too.*

Track Your Progress on The LEAN BODY, SMART LIFE App

The Archives

Click the QR Codes to Learn More Healthy Facts

Vegetable Archives

| Artichokes | Asparagus | Beets | Bok Choy | Broccolini |

| Brussels Sprouts | Cabbage | Carrots | Cauliflower | Edamame |

| Eggplant | Kale | Mushrooms | Okra | Peppers |

| Potatoes, Purple | Potatoes, Sweet | Radishes | Romanesco | Seaweed |

| Spinach | Squash: Zucchini, Butternut Squash | Sugar Snap Peas | Swiss Chard | Watercress |

Fruit Archives

Apples

Avocados

Black Berries

Blood Oranges

Cherries

Cranberries

Dates

Grapefruits

Grapes

Kiwis

Mangoes

Oranges

Papayas

Peaches

Pears

Pineapples

Pomegranates

Pumpkins

Raspberries

Watermelons

Grain Archives:

Barley

Black Rice

Buckwheat

Farro

Oatmeal

Popcorn

Quinoa Rice

Sorghum

Pulses (Dry Peas, Lentils and Beans) Archives:

Beans, Lentils

Garbanzo Beans

Pulses

Dairy & Egg Archives:

Cottage Cheese

Eggs

Greek Yogurt

Nuts & Seeds Archives:

Brazil Nuts

Chia Seeds

Flax Seeds

Peanuts

Hemp Seeds

Nuts

Herb & Spice Archives:

Cinnamon

Parsley

Turmeric

Seafood Archives:

Fish

Seafood

Flourless Peanut Butter Chocolate Swirl Cookies

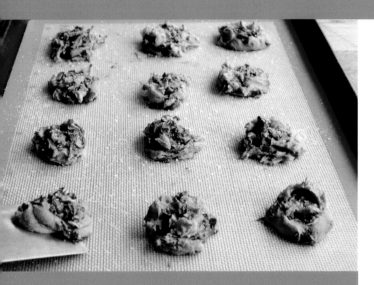

These yummy, moist cookies sweetened with raw honey are much healthier than a typical cookie. Beans replace the flour and egg while natural peanut butter is used instead of butter for an egg-, dairy-, and gluten-free dessert option. If people don't know they are healthy, no one will be the wiser! Wait until they rave before you spill the beans.

Ingredients

1 1/2 cups (or 1 can) chickpeas or white beans, well rinsed & patted dry

1 teaspoon vanilla extract

1/2 cup natural peanut butter

1/3 cup raw honey

1/4 teaspoon salt

2/3 cup semisweet chocolate chips

Nutritional Breakdown

1 cookie (1/16 of the recipe):
Protein 3.6 g, Fiber 2.1 g, Sodium 73.4 mg, Total fat 5.2 g, Saturated fat 0.8 g, Total carbs 7.2 g, Sugars 1.5 g, Calories 86 Kcal

Directions

Preheat your oven to 350°F.

Combine all the ingredients, except for the chocolate chips, in a food processor, and process until very smooth. Scrape the sides and process again until combined.

If the dough is warm after processing, mix in the chocolate chips as little as possible. These cookies look much more appealing if the chocolate isn't mixed all the way, but is lightly swirled. The mixture will be thick and sticky. Place sixteen spoonfuls of dough onto a cookie sheet lined with parchment paper.

If some chocolate chips have melted from the heat of the processor and the chocolate is already swirled through the cookie, bake for fifteen minutes. If the chocolate chips are all intact, place in a hot oven for two minutes, and then, using a toothpick, gently swirl the melted chocolate chips around the cookie. Continue to bake for thirteen more minutes and take it out after a total of fifteen minutes even if you think it's not done. Sprinkle hot cookies with one packet of monk fruit sugar substitute or stevia substitute if desired (optional).

Lemon Blueberry Yogurt Bread

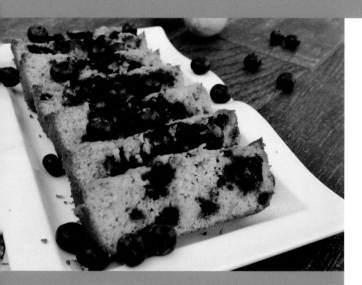

This yummy bread is healthy, and the yogurt makes it very moist. My friends frequently ask me for this recipe, and my family asks me to make it all the time. I love its refreshing taste, one that almost verges on a bread pudding. I always double this recipe and divide the batter among three loaf pans.

Ingredients

1 1/2 cups whole-wheat white flour

2 teaspoons baking powder

1/2 teaspoon salt

1 1/4 cups plain or vanilla nonfat Greek yogurt

1 cup pure maple syrup

2/3 to 3/4 cup sugar (depending on how sweet you want it)

3 extra large eggs

2 teaspoons grated lemon zest (2 small lemons)

1/2 teaspoon vanilla

1/4 cup canola oil

1 1/2 cup blueberries (frozen or fresh)

1/4 cup freshly squeezed lemon juice

2 tablespoons real maple syrup

Nutritional Breakdown

1/10 of this recipe:
Protein 7.4 g, Fiber 2.1 g, Sodium 146.7 mg, Total fat 7.5 g, Saturated fat 0.7 g, Total carbs 41.8 g, Sugars 22.8 g, Calories 245 Kcal

Directions

Preheat oven to 350°F. Grease one regular loaf pan and one mini loaf pan. If you double the recipe, use three loaf pans.

Stir together the flour, baking powder, and salt in a bowl. In another bowl, use a whisk or electric mixer to mix together the yogurt, sugar, 1/3 cup raw honey or real maple syrup, eggs, lemon zest, and vanilla. Slowly whisk the dry ingredients into the wet ingredients. With a rubber spatula, fold the oil into the batter. Gently fold in the blueberries. Pour the batter into the prepared loaf pans (about halfway full) and bake for about an hour or until a toothpick comes out clean.

Meanwhile, microwave the lemon juice and the 2 tablespoons real maple syrup in a microwave-safe bowl until dissolved.

When the bread is done, while the cake is still warm, poke several holes everywhere in the bread with a toothpick. Pour the lemon-syrup mixture over the bread evenly and allow it to soak in and cool completely before taking the bread out of the loaf pan.

Chapter 3: Eat Your Food

Visit FoodsWithJudes.com/book-content for recipes, articles and videos.

Video Games and Vegetables

When my kids were young, I had a rule: the only foods they could eat in the basement TV room were fruits and vegetables.

The rule lasted through their teenage years, and it went for the friends they brought home, too. My oldest son used to hang with his buddies at our house. These were teenage boys. They congregated in the basement to play serious video games and watch movies on the big screen. You might think they'd choose not to eat down there at all before they stooped to munching on vegetables. Nope.

"Mrs. Scharman!" the inevitable call came after a few minutes.

"Yes?" I called back.

"Can we have some fruits and vegetables?"

I pulled out two large, colorful plastic trays and some sugar snap peas, carrots, apples, peppers, and oranges. I chopped them up and poured everything I could find onto the trays in rainbow-colored formations, laughing to myself.

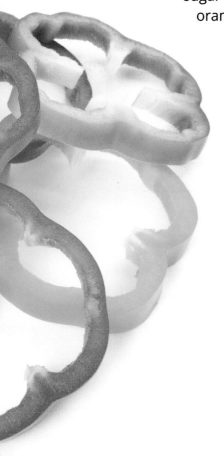

When the trays were piled high, I hollered, "Okay, come and get them!" Teenage feet came thundering up the stairs. The trays disappeared into the underground lair. They always came back completely empty.

Their veggie requests became a habit. This was wintertime in Cleveland, Ohio. My son and his friends spent a lot of time down there in that basement. And I can tell you, they ate a ton of fruits and vegetables along the way. Such a simple habit increased the amount of produce those boys ate during their teenage years and into their future. The simple changes you make to your surroundings can make a positive impact on your health!

Eat Up

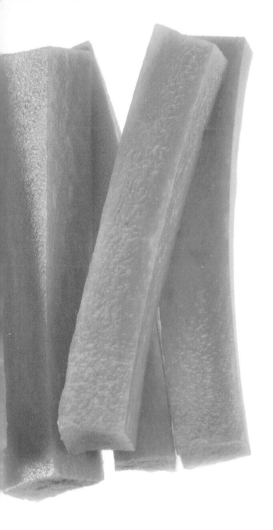

I know, I know. Whenever you buy fruits and vegetables, nobody eats them. They sit around and they go bad.

You're right—just having fruits and vegetables on the counter isn't enough. You can still find easy ways to get yourself and your family to eat healthy foods.

Buying healthy foods won't do you any good unless you eat them. Truckloads of critical vitamins, minerals, and phytonutrients might be sitting a few feet away from you every time you walk into your kitchen. Unless you come up with ways to close the gap between the counter and your stomach, your good intentions become useless.

That's why it's important to build some practical tricks and habits for transforming distant vegetables into food that you actually eat. Most of the time, that's easier to do than you might think.

66

...it's important to build some practical tricks and habits for transforming distant vegetables into food that you actually eat.

99

Vegetable Vanishing Act

When you eat food while you're doing other things, you eat more of it. That works against you if you're snacking on potato chips.

But it works in your favor if you're eating vegetables, especially if junk food is out-of-sight and unavailable.

The magic trick: if you cut it up and set it on a plate, someone will eat it. You can do this for yourself. Spend one or two minutes chopping up a vegetable that you wouldn't normally snack on. Then put it next to you while you're browsing the web. That vegetable will disappear. Magic.

The trick works for other people, too. Don't tell them that they have to eat what you're offering. Just set a plate of cut-up fruits and vegetables near them while they're doing other things. Just in case they get hungry. Again, those fruits and vegetables will magically disappear.

When I buy pears and leave them washed on the counter, no one eats them. I take ten seconds to cut a pear with an apple cutter and set the slices next to my kids, then voilà: the contents of the plate magically disappear. Kids will devour the fruits and vegetables without realizing it, just because they're there. Not only that, after a while they start to get used to them. They realize that those pears are actually delicious. And once in a while, who knows? You might even see them grabbing one from the fruit bowl or refrigerator. My young adult kids do almost every day now.

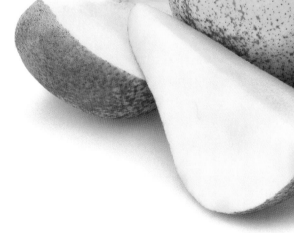

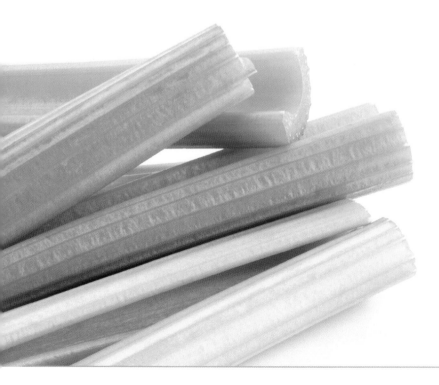

Office Wins

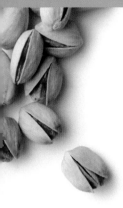

When it comes to eating healthy, the office has a way of sabotaging our good intentions. Someone brings in donuts. You work through lunch to make a deadline. The vending machine stares us in the face from where we're stationed in our desk chair.

Eating healthy at work may not be as easy as eating healthy at home. But with the right attitude and a few simple preparations, it can become a lot easier. Most work-friendly good-for-you snacks don't need a lot of prep. You just need to buy them and keep them with you. All you have to do is think ahead.

Raw nuts mixed with dried fruits such as blueberries and cranberries are great snacks to bring to work. In fact, pistachios with little mandarin oranges are some of my favorites. Any variety of nut is a healthy choice that keeps you full and adds extra protein, phytonutrients, vitamins, minerals, and good fats to your diet.

If you want a mid-morning snack, eat a low-sugar Greek yogurt to boost your protein intake.

Need Something Salty?

Skip the potato chips and try roasted seaweed snacks instead. They are full of flavor, and the tradeoff is only thirty nutritious calories. Roasted chickpeas are popping up in the stores. I like the Biena brand roasted chickpea snacks because they roast them instead of fry them. They are super crunchy, more so than when you make them at home, and they provide protein and fiber as well as other nutrients. Or for a sweet treat, bring along seasonal fruit such as small easy-to-peel oranges or a firm, crisp apple.

Challenge yourself to eat a piece of fruit every day at work as a snack. Set it on your desk and keep it in sight. Even if you aren't craving it, you'll eat it just because it's there. And if you can pair it with a protein food—such as peanut butter, nuts, a hard-boiled egg, roasted chickpeas, a mozzarella cheese stick, hummus, or yogurt—it will make it easier not to be tempted by the typical less-healthy office snacks. Every snack you eat should include a high-protein food and a fruit or vegetable: an orange and nuts, cottage cheese mixed with vegetables, pears with almond butter, or apples with peanut butter, to name a few. Try this, and not only will you feel better, but you'll concentrate better, too.

There are plenty of convenient whole-food snacks to take to the office. The key is picking healthy foods that you really enjoy and then making sure that you have them on hand. Over time, not only will you get used to them, but you'll enjoy them even more than those donuts, or anything you could buy from that vending machine, because of the way you feel after you eat them. You will recognize how much better you feel when you eat fruits and vegetables—and how poorly you feel by comparison when you resort to the workroom junk. Your tastes acclimate to less salt and sugar as well, so you're not as enticed, but the real trick is getting into the habit of having healthy food with you.

The Snack Box: Simple Snack Ideas

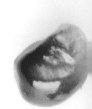

Frozen fruits make easy and delicious snacks. Mangoes from the frozen section are one of my favorites. Eat them straight out of the bag—like a healthy version of packaged candy. In fact, they are my nineteen-year-old daughter's favorite sweet snack. A couple of years ago, she got her whole tennis team eating them, and it was super easy for me to buy them, throw them into a cooler bag, and bring them to matches when it was our turn to bring the snack. You can try surprising everyone at work with mangoes instead of donuts. The tennis girls certainly liked the mangoes over donuts.

I love to nibble on pomegranate seeds and add them to my yogurt and hummus. You will never taste hummus the same way again. Use cucumbers to eat it instead of pita chips. Fresh pomegranate seeds come out so easily when you hit the pomegranate with a wooden spoon.

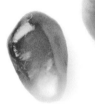

People also swear by frozen grapes. When my bananas start to turn brown, I peel them, chop them into slices, and freeze them. Then I eat them plain or with a dab of natural peanut butter.

 Pomegranate Magic: Seeds Out, No Mess

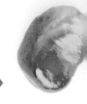

Feeling Energetic?

Toss some frozen bananas into a food processor with some strawberries, almond butter, or cocoa. Let it blend until it's the consistency of soft-serve. It will satisfy your ice cream cravings—the healthy way!

Dates are another great option. Eat them plain, or stuff them with cheese, nut butter, or nuts to make a filling snack or a decadent appetizer. Fresh figs are amazing too.

Limed apples or apples with natural peanut butter make a filling snack. My kids never used to like apples; once the slices started to turn brown, they wouldn't touch them. After I started squeezing lime juice over the apple slices, they miraculously started to love them. I also enjoy hummus with cucumbers, red peppers, or celery. Edamame, yogurt, Wasa Light Rye crackers topped with cottage cheese and cucumbers, and pistachio nuts in their shells are on my go-to list as well.

Popcorn is Another Simple, Healthy Snack

I'm not talking about microwave popcorn or theater popcorn (which is loaded with so many calories that it's like eating a pound of ribs topped with a scoop of ice cream). Popcorn is entirely whole grain, with plenty of antioxidants, fiber, and manganese. The key is making sure it's made with less fat that is better for you. Organic light popcorn is everywhere in stores now, if you want it already popped.

Put a handful of popcorn kernels in a paper lunch bag, fold down the top edge, and microwave it until you hear three to five seconds inbetween pops. A hot air popcorn popper works too. Trade out the butter by spraying olive oil infused with lime or other flavors onto the popped kernels. Get creative with spices such as garlic powder, smoked paprika, turmeric, or chili powder. Or for a sweeter option, drizzle cocoa powder and either pure maple syrup or raw honey over popped popcorn.

Check Out My Healthy Popcorn Recipes

The healthy-snack possibilities are endless – and so are the health benefits.

Three Magic Tricks

Those of us who live with picky eaters know how hard it is to get people to eat their vegetables. Sometimes it feels like an impossible challenge. However, there are a few simple ways to get your kids (and everyone else who is leery of vegetables) to increase their healthy food intake.

Pre-Meal Vegetable Platter

When kids (both big and small) complain that they're hungry, don't let them make a beeline for the pantry. Tell them that they can eat any of the vegetables on the table, but that's it. Be consistent. It's either the vegetables or nothing. They make the choice, so it's not a power struggle. They choose to eat their vegetables. If you want them to try something new, put it on the vegetable plate. People are a lot more likely to try new things when they're at their hungriest, and when they don't feel like they're being forced to eat them.

This doesn't mean you have to put a lot of extra time and effort into cutting things up. You can buy vegetables that are already cut, or vegetables that don't need much cutting. Sugar snap peas, baby carrots, and grape tomatoes pour right onto the plate. Cucumbers and red peppers are quick and easy to cut. Whatever you choose, I recommend having more than one type of vegetable out there so that people have more choices and more exposure. Hummus or salad dressing may be nice encouragement at first, but as time goes on and eating vegetables becomes a habit, you can skip the dressing altogether, and the veggies will still get eaten.

This is a great chance to introduce new vegetables with no pressure to eat them. Routinely add an unfamiliar vegetable to the mix without mentioning it. You may be surprised about what gets eaten.

Serve Vegetables First at Mealtimes

This habit can make a huge difference to your family's vegetable intake. If you serve vegetables first at mealtimes, people will eat more of them. Why? Because they're hungrier at the start of the meal than they are at the end of it. Don't put anything on the table to compete with your vegetable. The salad or the broccoli goes on there first and alone. Add the other food only after the vegetable is gone.

Eat Only Fruits and Vegetables While Doing Activities

We eat more when we're doing other things. So we may as well eat more fruits and vegetables. Snacks are a prime time to get fruits and vegetables into kids and adults alike. Use them to replace crackers and chips. Chop them up and make them available. As long as there's no processed food competition, the fruits and veggies will disappear.

Consistent guidelines or rules help, too. Make a family rule that only fruits and vegetables can be eaten in common areas such as the TV or game room, and all other foods have to be eaten in the kitchen, sitting at the table. A rule like this is a great strategy for supporting a healthy weight in children. Not only are you eating more healthy food, but you're also eating less unhealthy food at the same time. Like my son's friends in the TV room, with a rule like this in place, people will eat fruits and vegetables without thinking twice.

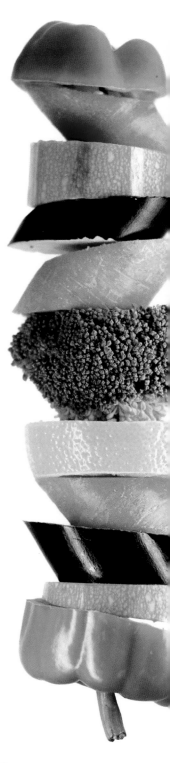

 Lose Weight by Tricking Your Brain

FIX #4

Rearrange Your Environment

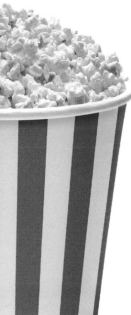

Most of us eat without thinking. If it's there, we eat it. The more food that happens to be near us, the more we will eat. We don't eat food because we're hungry, we eat it because it's available. And that has disastrous consequences for our weight and our health.

Rather than fight our willpower to counter excess pounds, we can change our surroundings. It's a bit like tricking our brains to eliminate decisions that add on the pounds. We can at least make these poor food decisions less convenient. Rearranging our stomping grounds prevents us from feeling deprived because we're taking away the temptation before it begins. This leads to greater success in our battle to eat better.

Our environments make a huge impact on how much food we eat and what type of food we eat. Brian Wansink, PhD, director of the Cornell Food and Brand Lab, has conducted hundreds of research studies examining the cues that make us eat. He and his team have discovered that the more we can eat, the more we do eat.

 # Think About It.

For example, one study presented people who had just eaten at a restaurant with free movie tickets. The tickets included popcorn and a drink. Participants were given five-day-old stale popcorn that tasted like Styrofoam. Some were given large buckets, and others were given medium-sized buckets. None of them were hungry, and the food wasn't good. By the end of the movie, the people with the big buckets of popcorn had eaten 34 percent more popcorn than the participants with smaller buckets had eaten.

They Had More Food, So They Ate More Food

You can change your environment around to eat less bad food, and more good food. The strategies are simple. Yet they make a big difference!

Use smaller plates and bowls. Wansink found that smaller plates can lead us to think that we're eating more food than we really are. The same is true with glasses. Tall, narrow glasses make us feel like we're drinking more. Shorter, wider ones give us the feeling of drinking less. Use the tall ones for less healthful drinks, so you take in less. The color of your plate can also affect how much you eat. Wansink's team discovered that those whose plates were a similar color to their food served themselves 18 percent more food than did those with opposite-colored plates.

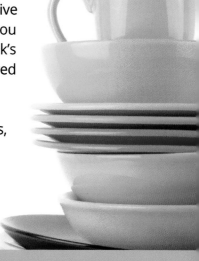

Your surroundings also affect how often you eat. In one of Wansink's studies, administrative assistants with a bowl of candy on their desks ate an average of nine pieces per day and weighed 15.4 pounds more than those who kept the candy bowl six feet away and ate only four pieces a day, as well as those who ate less because they couldn't see it at all.

Did You Know?

Dr. Wansink found we are three times more likely to eat the first thing we see when we open a cupboard or the refrigerator than we are to eat the fifth thing we see. You can imagine how much more likely we are to eat food out on the counter. One of his studies reported that women who kept even one box of cereal on the counter were twenty-five pounds heavier than their neighbors who kept all cereal out of sight.

Fruits and vegetables hidden in the crisper should be moved to eye level, and less-healthy food should be stored in harder-to-see places in opaque containers or foil. Store unhealthy foods out of sight, in inconvenient places, but keep healthy foods in sight and in reach.

If the off-limit food stays at the grocery store, all the better. If it manages to make its way into the cart, store it in an annoying place in the house, such as the garage or the storage room. I've moved my chocolate chips from the pantry to the downstairs storage room several times because I realized I was grabbing unnecessary handfuls more often than I would if I didn't see them on the shelf. Out of sight, out of mind. The more effort it takes to get to the bad food, the less likely you are to eat it.

Fruits and vegetables hidden in the crisper should be moved to eye level, and less-healthy food should be stored in harder-to-see places in opaque containers or foil. Store unhealthy foods out of sight, in inconvenient places, but keep healthy foods in sight and in reach.

Think About It.

Once you've served the green salad and vegetables at dinner, serve portioned food on the plates rather than serving "family style." Dr. Wansink's team found this strategy helps us to eat 19 percent less food. If you have to use serving bowls, be sure to take them off the table after everyone's first helping—except for the fruits and vegetables! When food is in reach, we eat more of it. A family-style dinner, where everything is in reach, promotes overeating.

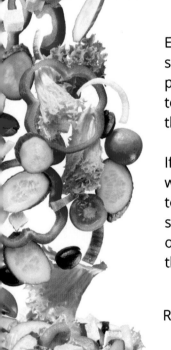

Eating out of large packages leads to eating more than if you have a smaller package, so dish your food into a small cup. Better yet, repackage food into single-serving portions. Bigger packages also encourage us to cook 22 percent more food, according to another study headed by Dr. Wansink. That's okay if you put half the food away in the refrigerator or freezer for another meal before you serve up.

If you tend to eat while you do other activities such as surfing the web, reading, or watching TV, you may want to think again. Taking your mind away from paying attention to your food means that you eat without thinking. Hopefully, you have served up a single serving and put the package or food away because you aren't cognizant of what or how much you are taking in. Conversing with others in person is about the only thing you should be doing while you are eating, to avoid mindlessly eating too much.

Reengineering your environment with these simple but powerful strategies will make positive change happen without you even realizing it's happening. The biggest problem is telling yourself these changes are so small they couldn't possibly make a difference, so you don't make them. In fact, as small as they are, they make a difference over time. Because these aren't hard changes that make you feel deprived, it is easy to make them real habits that last.

The other problem is thinking that because you know certain habits cause you to eat more of the wrong foods, you won't allow that to happen. It's not that easy, because many of these things are subconscious illusions or brain tricks. Even the researchers knowing the results of these bad habits couldn't change the outcomes. Knowledge isn't enough in this case. Because these small changes don't test your willpower or make you feel deprived, why not implement them in your life?

Fix #4 Action Plan:

✓ *Eat without distractions such as computers, TV or reading.*

✓ *Start with a small amount of food.*

✓ *Use small plates, bowls, & spoons.*

✓ *Drink everything that isn't water from tall, narrow glasses.*

✓ *Keep unhealthy and neutral foods out of sight or in an inconvenient place.*

✓ *Place healthy foods in plain sight.*

✓ *Eat packaged foods in small servings. If you buy large packages, divide them into smaller packages right after the purchase.*

✓ *Keep serving dishes (except for salad and vegetables) off the dining table after everyone has been served.*

✓ *Eat only part of a snack, and then wait ten to fifteen minutes. This smaller amount may be enough to satisfy you.*

✓ *Keep unhealthy food out of sight and out of reach in the office, and keep fruits and vegetables in sight and in reach.*

✓ *Avoid family-style eating with too many choices. (Unless it's vegetables—in that case, bring it on!)*

✓ *Avoid buffet-style restaurants at all times.*

Track Your Progress on The LEAN BODY, SMART LIFE App

Turkish Hummus

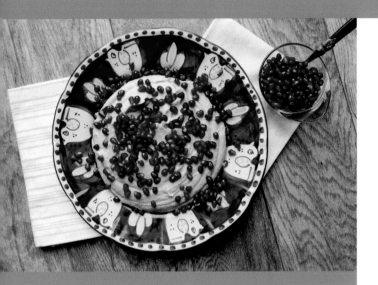

I learned how to make this hummus when I lived in the Middle East and took a Turkish cooking class with my husband. The food was delicious, and I've been making this hummus ever since. Pomegranate seeds add a burst of juicy sweetness that makes this hummus surprisingly wonderful.

Ingredients

4 cans cooked organic chickpeas or 6 cups cooked chickpeas

1 cup tahini (sesame tahini)

1/2 teaspoon baking soda

1 teaspoon minced garlic (or more to taste)

4 tablespoons oil

1/2 cup lemon juice (or more to taste)

1 1/2 teaspoon salt (more to taste)

1 teaspoon cumin powder

1/4 cup cold water

6–8 tablespoons plain yogurt

For Garnish: (optional)

2–3 tablespoons olive oil

paprika

pomegranate seeds

Nutritional Breakdown

For 4 tablespoons:

Protein 5.7 g, Fiber 3.9 g, Sodium 157 mg, Fat 5.9 g, Saturated fat 0.7 g, Total carbs 16.1 g, Sugars 2.8 g, Calories 132 Kcal

Directions

Rinse the canned chickpeas with water. Transfer them to a saucepan. Add baking soda and water to cover the chickpeas. Bring to a boil and simmer at a soft boil for thirty to forty minutes. Turn the heat off and cool.

Put the chickpeas in a food processor. Add the remaining ingredients and process until smooth. Chill in the fridge for two to three hours before serving.

Spread it in a shallow serving dish, swirling it with the back of a spoon, pour olive oil in the center, and sprinkle with paprika or top with pomegranate seeds. Serve with cucumbers and whole grain pita bread. Refrigerate up to four days, and then freeze.

Avocado Black Bean Corn Salad

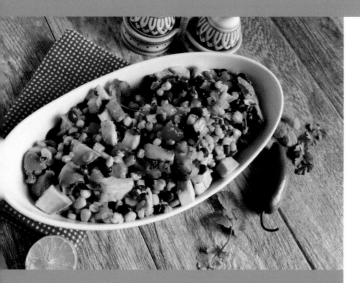

This salad is one of my most requested recipes. It is easy to make and very healthy. The sweetness of the fruit salsa offsets the tartness of freshly squeezed lime juice, without adding sugar.

Ingredients

2 cans black beans, rinsed well and drained

1 16-oz. bag frozen roasted corn (3 1/2 cups)

2 cups mango, peach, or pineapple salsa

1/2 cup fresh lime juice (4 limes)

4 avocados, diced

1/4 cup chopped red onion, chopped fine

salt to taste

1/2 cup cilantro

Nutritional Breakdown

For 1/15 of this recipe (about 1/2 cup):

Protein 3.4 g, Fiber 4.6 g, Sodium 135.6 mg, Fat 4.9 g, Saturated fat 0.5 g, Total carbs 14.4 g, Sugars 4.4 g, Calories 127 Kcal

Directions

Mix black beans, frozen corn, and fruit salsa together in a medium bowl. Squeeze the limes and set aside. Add the avocado to the salad, and before mixing, immediately add the lime juice, red onion, and salt to the salad. Gently mix all ingredients together. Feel free to give this salad a little kick with some hot pepper flakes or hot sauce. A freshly diced jalapeño pepper tastes great too. Add the cilantro prior to serving.

Chapter 4: Track Your Food

Visit FoodsWithJudes.com/book-content for recipes, articles and videos.

Twenty-Four Raw Almonds

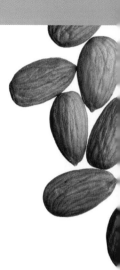

What fills you up, keeps you feeling full, and appears to have almost no weight-gain effect?

The Answer Is Twenty-Four Raw Almonds

Twenty-four raw almonds make about one ounce or 1/4 cup of nuts. Researchers have been studying almonds and have found intriguing results. Several studies have indicated that almond snacks seem to promote weight loss when up against lower-calorie, high-carb snacks. Almonds reduce appetite, steady blood sugars, fight heart disease, and help reduce chronic inflammation.

Did You Know?

The research indicates that although almonds and almond butter are high in calories, they don't seem to contribute to weight gain. One study at Purdue University looked at the effects of adding 360 calories or two ounces of almonds to participants' daily diets. After ten weeks, the almond eaters experienced no significant weight change. The researchers concluded that the almond intake made the participants feel full so that they ate fewer calories at other meals. They also found that some calories from almonds pass through your body unabsorbed, so they can't be stored as fat.

The Bottom Line

People who eat twenty-four to forty-eight raw almonds for snacks are less hungry. They stay full longer. And they are less likely to gain weight. Even better, almonds are a terrific way to add nutrient-rich protein to your diet.

Now, if you eat a whole bag of almonds, you may gain weight. But if you count out twenty-four almonds, put them in a container or bag, and take them to work with you every day, you're home free. They don't seem to cost your body any calories at all.

Maybe there's no such thing as a free lunch. But when you track your almonds, there may be such a thing as a free snack.

On Track for Success

Building small, healthy habits is the optimal way to make big changes to your health. An important way to build those habits is to track your changes.

Simple, easy tracking is a supportive tool. And while you're getting into the habit of eating healthy, it's an indispensable one. Tracking is important to the psychology of how we approach our wellness. We use it to see where we're at and to motivate ourselves to keep moving forward. We can use it to keep ourselves accountable for what we eat—without stressing ourselves out too much.

Tracking shouldn't be a big and scary undertaking. Don't look at it as an all-or-nothing proposition. Your health isn't a huge one-time challenge that you put a lot of energy into at first and then quit. Good health should be easy, and tracking should be simple, not overwhelming.

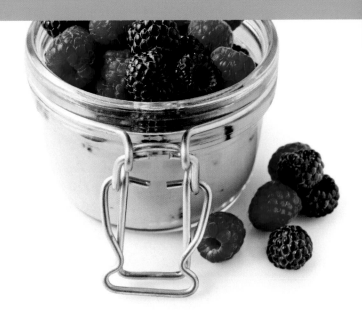

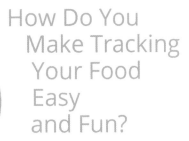

How Do You Make Tracking Your Food Easy and Fun?

First, track only the positive progress you make. The idea here isn't to punish yourself for breaking the rules. The idea is to reward yourself for making good choices. If you eat an apple and a piece of cake, don't chew yourself out for eating the cake. Track that apple, and congratulate yourself for increasing your fruit intake, because even one extra apple will help you. Positive psychology will take you a long way.

Second, start simple. Choose from the suggested fixes the LEAN BODY, SMART LIFE app recommends you focus on the fixes your struggle with most. Or choose from the list of twelve fixes in this book. You can add as many fixes as you want to track on the app, but only a maximum of three fixes show up on the home screen at one time. That helps you to really concentrate on your focus fix. Even though it's tempting, don't take on too many fixes at once. Tracking is meant to help you get into the groove of a new way of living. However, too many things to focus on can derail your efforts!

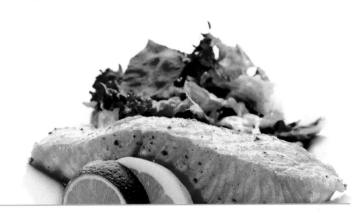

Third, tell someone else what you're doing. Many studies have reported that when you start a new behavior, it's more likely to stick if you share your progress with others. You care what they think about your efforts, and that makes you more accountable. The LEAN BODY, SMART LIFE app allows you to share your progress with another person, such as a friend, coworker, or registered dietitian nutritionist.

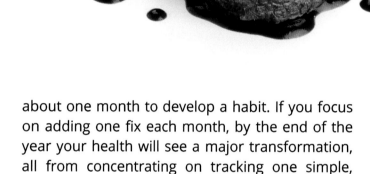

> ❝
>
> Many studies have reported that when you start a new behavior, it's more likely to stick if you share your progress with others.
>
> ❞

Keep tracking until you've developed the habit. You need to do something for only twenty-eight days before it becomes habitual. Once you find yourself automatically thinking, "Oh, I need to have more vegetables with this meal so I'm eating about half of my meal in veggies," you know that tracking those vegetables has been effective. You can keep tracking vegetables even though you're now subconsciously aware of eating them, but you can start focusing on tracking something else too. There are twelve fixes in this book, and it takes only

about one month to develop a habit. If you focus on adding one fix each month, by the end of the year your health will see a major transformation, all from concentrating on tracking one simple, easy fix at a time.

Push forward and expose yourself to each fix by adding a new fix to focus on each week for twelve weeks. After trying out each fix, you will have a good idea of what fixes you may want to add going forward for a month at a time to establish each habit. The LEAN BODY, SMART LIFE app will suggest fixes helpful to your individual struggles and help you track your fixes for optimal success.

Tracking reminds you that your health isn't something you stop and start. Your health is something you do mindfully.

Your health is something you can enjoy.

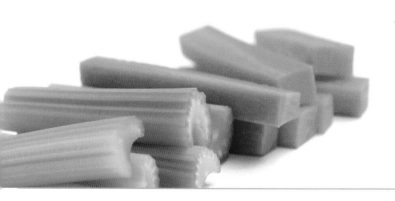

Don't Count Calories

Tracking Does Not Mean Counting Calories

I purposely choose not to count calories. Calories are like the gas in a car; the quality of the gas you put in affects how your body runs. Your body uses different types of calories differently. At the end of the day, the total number of calories we eat is less important than the type of calories we take in.

More than that, tracking calories has a negative effect on your psychology. This isn't a diet. Yes, you're going to lose fat weight, but this is actually a lifestyle and a new way of thinking.

There is a balance to strike between being careful and overdoing it. Too much tracking can make you feel deprived—especially when you track calories. When that happens, you lose your motivation, and it often makes you want to drop the whole thing.

Even with the things you do track, never be so strict with yourself that you feel like you're on a diet. Track things until they become habits that you feel comfortable doing most of the time. That's right—**most** of the time. Remember, this is a lifestyle. If you do the twelve fixes in this book 75 percent of the time for the rest of your life, that's better than doing just a few fixes 99 percent of the time for three months and then abandoning them like you would a diet.

The more little things you do over the long term, the more your health will benefit down the line, not to mention your present feelings of accomplishment, alertness, and energy. Don't count calories. Do count positive choices. And do celebrate the efforts you make to improve your health!

There Are Plenty of Ways To Do Your Tracking

 Think About It

The most obvious way to track is to write it down on paper. Keep a food journal that's small enough to carry around. Buy a day planner and use it for food instead of appointments. Studies have shown that the act of writing down what you eat and drink makes you more aware of what you're consuming, which helps you make better food choices. According to a study by Kaiser Permanente's Center for Health Research looking at seventeen hundred people trying to lose weight across the United States, people who kept daily food records six days a week lost about twice as much as did those who kept a log only one day a week or less.

Do Your Tracking Digitally

Note your foods eaten on your smartphone or tablet. Better yet, use the LEAN BODY, SMART LIFE app, designed to help you track all of the twelve fixes introduced in this 12-FIX LEAN LIFE PLAN. This very simple app helps you concentrate on the fixes you choose to track without complicating the matter by unnecessarily tracking calories and other food components that make it seem more like a diet and detract from your health-promoting goals. This app is easy to use, making it simple to share your progress with your friends and to view your trends over time.

Some people make it even easier by just tracking their food with pictures. If you have a smartphone, the camera is always in your pocket, and the device does your date keeping for you. Just snap a picture of the food you eat that pertains to the fix you have chosen to improve.

When it comes to tracking methods, there is just one rule: do whatever is easiest for you. The last thing you want is for tracking to get overwhelming. When that happens, it hurts you more than it helps you. Keep your methods simple and fun. Tracking the fixes on the LEAN BODY, SMART LIFE app is easier than keeping a detailed food diary, and you'll be willing to do it for longer.

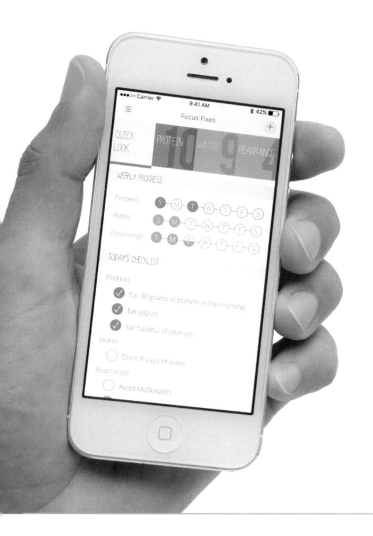

When it comes to tracking methods, there is just one rule: do whatever is easiest for you.

Track Your Fruits and Vegetables

Looking for a good place to start tracking? Fueling your body with fruits and vegetables makes a fantastic first step.

Try to eat a fruit or vegetable every time you eat. Did you make them half of your meals and snacks? This is a good way to start tracking your fruit and vegetable intake. If you can make fruits and vegetables about 50 percent of all your meals and snacks, you will make a huge improvement to your health, especially over the long haul.

After you get used to eating more fruits and vegetables, challenge yourself to go even further. Try for a variety of kinds and colors to boost your intake of nutrients. Dark leafy greens, cooked tomatoes, and anything that's a rich yellow, orange, purple, or red color is ideal. Seriously, your body will rejoice at the nutrients you are putting into it.

 The Daily "Detox Cleanse" for Life

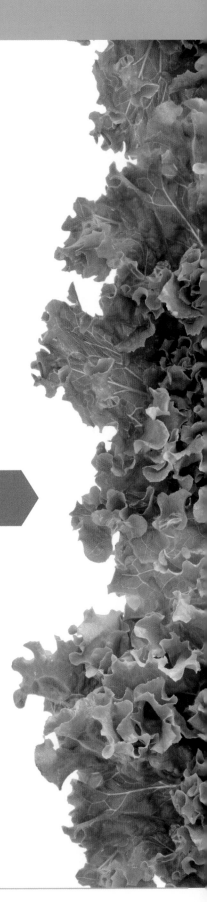

FIX #5

Make Fruits and Vegetables 50 Percent of Your Meals and Snacks

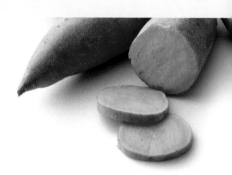

Don't set this fix aside just because you've heard people tell you to eat more fruits and vegetables a million times. There's a reason you hear it over and over! This is one of the most important fixes you can make for your health.

Fruits and vegetables deliver thousands of phytonutrients that are extremely powerful. The Dietary Inflammatory Index (DII) rated the nutrients in fruits and vegetables among the highest, having some of the greatest impact in fighting and repairing damage throughout the body.

Phytonutrients in fruits and vegetables serve as antioxidants to help cells stay healthy and repair DNA damage caused by smoking and other factors such as pollution, poor diet patterns, alcohol, and other harmful toxins. Eating plenty of fruits and vegetables gives a tremendous boost to your immune system and has been identified as a critical factor in disease prevention.

Following this fix could even help you live longer. A meta-analysis of 95 studies looking at fruit and vegetable intake found that 7.8 million premature deaths in the world could be avoided if people ate 800 grams of fruits and vegetables a day. For reference, one medium apple alone is about 182 grams. Think about eating fruits and vegetables as your daily "detox cleanse."

Our brains benefit from eating lots of fruits and vegetables too. Research has indicated that phytonutrients protect brain tissue from breaking down to promote quicker and sharper cognitive skills. Specifically, vitamins C and E may aid neurons in the brain to communicate better with each other.

Vitamin A appears to boost the brain's ability to switch from one mental activity to another. Certain phytonutrients, including anthocyanins that are in deep red and blue colored produce, appear to decrease inflammation in the brain, improve brain signals, and improve blood flow to the brain.

Eating more fruits and vegetables enhances weight loss, lowers blood pressure, decreases heart disease and cancer, offers illness protection, and promotes clearer thinking. There's no question: fruits and vegetables are the biggest bang for your health!

Make fruits and vegetables half of the food you eat. That goes for both meals and snacks. Remember that french fries don't count as vegetables. Replace white potatoes with purple potatoes and sweet potatoes as often as you can. Beans and lentils are also on this vegetable list, along with starchy vegetables.

Try to include a variety of fruits and vegetables in your diet, and find new ways of preparing the ones you're used to eating. The less boring they are, the more you'll eat them!

Fix #5 Action Plan:

✓ *Make fruits and vegetables half of all your meals and snacks.*

✓ *Pair nuts with a piece of fruit and take them with you for a snack.*

✓ *Bring fruits or vegetables with you everywhere you go.*

✓ *Keep cut-up vegetables and fruit at eye level in the refrigerator.*

✓ *Try roasting your vegetables (chapter 8).*

✓ *Make extra vegetables, including lentils and beans, to mix with whole grains all week.*

✓ *Place cut-up vegetables and fruit within arm's length.*

✓ *Place a plate of cut-up vegetables out for those who are hungry prior to a meal.*

✓ *Adopt a policy for you and your family of eating only fruits and vegetables while participating in activities such as surfing the net, checking email, reading, or watching TV.*

Track Your Progress on The LEAN BODY, SMART LIFE App

Track Your Protein

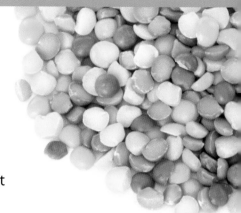

Protein is probably the most critical nutrient to track. Not only does it help keep you full longer with fewer cravings, but you need protein to prevent age-related muscle loss, build new muscle, and promote optimal health. Protein foods from plants (such as beans, dried peas, lentils, nuts, seeds, and quinoa) as well as from yogurt, kefir, seafood, cottage cheese (the highest source of leucine for building muscles), and even barnyard eggs have the greatest health-promoting potential. But how much protein should you get, and when should you get it?

According to Donald Layman, PhD, professor emeritus of nutrition at the University of Illinois, we need about 30 grams of protein in one meal to stimulate muscle building. However, more than 50 grams of protein per meal is too much and doesn't benefit our muscles.

Aim to take in about 30 grams of high-quality protein each meal for a total of about 90 grams (or at least 75 grams) of protein spread throughout the day. Of course, some of those 90 grams can be included in your snacks to help you boost your intake.

This may seem like a lot of protein, but it is actually considered a moderate protein intake. Those 90 grams of protein amount to only 360 calories—only 18 percent of a typical two-thousand-calorie diet. The Institute of Medicine recommends that you get 10 to 35 percent of your calories from protein, so 90 grams is even at the lower end of that range.

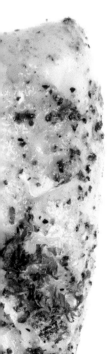

To be more specific to your body size, multiply your current weight in pounds by 0.6, and that will give you an estimated number of grams of protein you need per day to promote body fat loss while building muscle: 175 lbs. × 0.6 = 105 grams of protein per day.

Use a factor of 0.7 instead of 0.6 if you want greater fat loss, if you're greater than sixty-five years old, or if you participate in intense exercise for more than an hour a day: 175 lbs. × 0.7 = 122 grams of protein per day.

Track your protein the way you track everything else: focus on the fix but don't be too meticulous and make yourself crazy. Everyone is different, and these numbers are just estimates. Try to eat healthy protein throughout the day, but especially in the morning. Include protein sources such as Greek yogurt, eggs, beans, lentils, dried peas, nuts, seeds, or fish at each meal and snack spread out evenly during the day. Use less meat, pork, or poultry.

How Much Protein Are You Eating?

Use this handy chart to help you track your protein intake.

Type of Food	Protein Content	Type of Food	Protein Content
1 egg	6 g	1/2 cup shelled edamame	11 g
1 cup cottage cheese	28 g	1 1/8 cups edamame pods	11 g
1 cup greek yogurt	20 g	1 cup tofu	20 g
1 cup yogurt	11 g	1/2 cup dry roasted soybeans	34 g
1 oz. mozzarella	7 g	1/2 cup pumkin seeds	6 g
1 string cheese	6 g	1/2 cup amaranth	13 g
2 tbsp peanut butter	8 g	1/2 cup buckwheat	11 g
1/2 cup walnuts	6 g	1 cup cooked quinoa	9 g
1/2 cup almonds	10 g	3 tbsp shelled hemp seeds	10 g
1/2 cup peanuts	17 g	1 lean sausage link	9 g
1 cup milk	8 g	3 oz. chicken	26 g
1 cup soy milk	8 g	3 oz. salmon	22 g
1 oz. cheddar cheese	7 g	3 oz. cod	19 g
1 cup oatmeal	6 g	3 oz. shrimp	17 g
1/2 cup cooked lentils	9 g	3 oz. pork	22 g
1/2 cup white beans	9 g	3 oz. lean beef	21 g
1/2 cup black beans	8 g		

Whole Grains for More Daily Detox

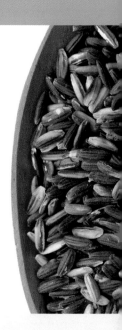

Dietary fiber found in whole grains, (such as oats, brown or black rice, sorghum, farro, quinoa, barley, popcorn, and whole wheat) fruits, and vegetables are ranked among the strongest components of food to fight chronic inflammation in the Dietary Inflammatory Index. It appears that the fiber ferments during digestion and produces a fatty acid that blocks inflammation. This type of fiber is particularly high in whole grains, dry beans, and peas.

Carbs, and wheat in particular, have been demonized by the media. Sugar and refined flour (typically white flour) deserve their bad rap. These processed carbs are associated with chronic disease, mental decline, and depression. Whole grains that haven't been refined and stripped of valuable nutrients and bulk are haphazardly thrown into the pot.

 ## Think About It.

We need health-benefiting whole grains for longer-lasting fuel for energy, for both our bodies and our brains. Our muscles need to keep stored energy in them so we are energized to move. Our brains are more mentally alert and focused throughout the day when we eat whole grains. The fiber and phytonutrients in whole grains help release glucose slowly into the bloodstream, providing a steady supply of energy to your body and brain.

Whole grains have a plethora of research revealing their many health benefits. Beyond helping to control blood sugar, these undefiled grains lower the risk of type 2 diabetes, heart disease, blood pressure, and cancer. Not only do whole grains help control weight, but eating them instead of refined, processed grains cuts down on the amount of body fat around your middle.

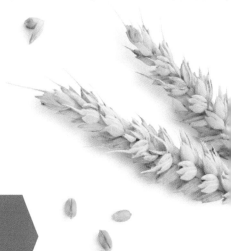

 Your Carb Sweet Spot: Ideal Carb Intake for Weight Loss

FIX #6

Eat Between Three and Six Servings of Whole Grains per Day

Eat at least three servings of whole grains per day, but no more than six servings. Three servings is the absolute minimum; don't be tempted to skip them. You need those three servings to lose fat weight and better your health. Remember, I'm talking about whole grains that are filled with thousands of phytonutrients, fiber, vitamins, and minerals that truly make a difference to your energy level, thinking power, inflammation level, disease state, and gut health. Taking whole grains out of your diet completely is analogous to taking vegetables out of your diet. But because some people demonize all carbs, the true power of whole grains is often lost.

Eating whole grains helps you increase your muscle and improve your body composition. These nutritious calories from whole grains are used as fuel to get the most out your movement throughout the day. They protect your muscles from being broken down for energy and to protect the protein you eat, so it is used to repair and build more muscle.

More than six servings may be too much if you want to lose weight. For those engaging in moderate exercise less than an hour per day and are of average to small build, this three to six serving range should be about right.

If you're doing intense exercise, of course, you may need more. If you are a large person or are in athletic training, you will almost certainly need more than six servings of whole grains. If you aren't in training, you still may need to increase your servings of whole grains if you require more energy to exercise strenuously on any given day.

One serving of whole grain is about half a cup or one slice of whole grain bread. Keep track of the number of slices and servings of whole grains foods you eat every day. As long as you stay within the range of three to six whole grain servings per day, you will be doing well.

Put the emphasis on ancient grains, but be sure to track all the whole grains you eat. Of course, when you eat a refined, processed grain, such as white bread or white rice, rather than a whole grain on occasion, the refined grain should be counted as part of the three to six grains you eat each day. But do know you are replacing foods that actually help you decrease your body fat, absorb fewer calories than refined carbs, fight disease, and keep your mind alert with foods that increase your body fat and contribute to illness and grogginess.

Even though three to six servings of whole grains may be less than what you're used to eating, this is not a low-carbohydrate plan. Fruits and vegetables are great sources of carbohydrates, and vegetables such as beans and lentils are very filling. Also, whole grains are more satisfying than processed grains, so you can count your grains and not worry about going hungry!

For a complete rundown of some of the healthiest whole grains you can eat, refer to the Grain Archives in Chapter 2. To learn how to easily prepare these delicious grains, refer to Chapter 8.

Fix #6 Action Plan:

✓ *Eat three to six whole-grain 1/2-cup servings per day.*

✓ *Include ancient grains as a part of your daily whole grain intake.*

✓ *Count your whole-grain servings correctly: one serving of cooked whole grains is about half a cup or one piece of bread.*

✓ *Try preparing and eating one new whole grain every month.*

✓ *Try mixing unfamiliar whole grains with familiar grains such as rice.*

✓ *Cook extra whole grains and use them throughout the week. They stay good in the refrigerator for five days.*

✓ *Sourdough whole-grain bread made with a long fermentation time is the healthiest bread choice. During those times you eat white bread, at least choose a sourdough bread variety.*

✓ *Thinly sliced whole-grain bread allows you to have two slices per serving. For example, Dave's Killer Bread offers tasty thin-sliced whole grain varieties.*

Track Your Progress on The LEAN BODY, SMART LIFE App

Track in Groups

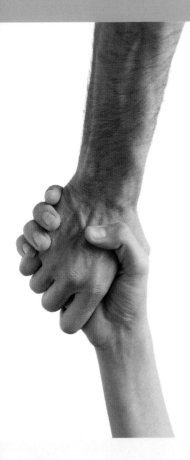

Tracking With Others Gives You Accountability

Do you need help to begin tracking? Track your fixes with a group of people.

If you have no one to answer to but yourself, you're more likely to let things slide. Sharing your goals and results with a friend or coworker gives you stronger motivation to keep yourself on track.

Anything is more fun when you can socialize with other people along the way. And the more fun you have, the more successful you are.

Tracking in a group can be easy. Get together and discuss which fix you want to track first. Then come together once a week and share your progress. You don't even have to do it in person. Email, Facebook, and online group chats work, too. In fact, the LEAN BODY, SMART LIFE app lets you share your progress with others.

 ## Think About It.

You can put a group together at the office. You can start one with the other parents on the playground. You can get your family on board. Research shows that making a lifestyle change in the company of other people keeps your motivation and your spirits up.

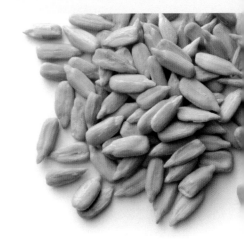

When I help companies with their wellness programs, the employees pick something that they are willing to track together, as a team. One team member is in charge of tabulating everyone's tracking results. Often, they choose to track one of the twelve fixes every month, allowing each person about thirty days to form a new habit. The team members decide together how they want to track, and the team leader encourages all of them to track their progress and post the results to help everyone get involved. That's what I call teamwork!

Butternut Squash Kale Farro Pilaf

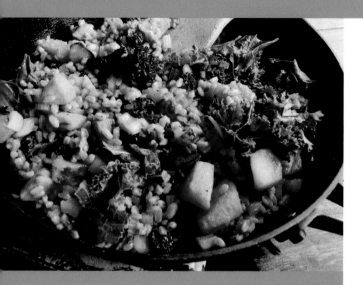

The combination of roasted butternut squash, hearty farro, dried sweetened cranberries, crunchy celery, and sturdy yet tender kale makes for a delicious winter dish that's easy and pretty. The curry and coriander flavors are even better the next day, so it's perfect for leftovers. Unlike spinach, the kale holds up for a few days, although it does shrink. Just add more kale prior to reheating to add even more powerful nutrition.

Ingredients

2/3 cup uncooked semi-pearled farro (1 1/2 cups cooked)

1 1/2 teaspoon ground cumin, divided

2 cups butternut squash, peeled and diced in 1/2" cubes

1 to 2 cups kale, torn from stem in bite-sized pieces (don't include stem)

1/2 cup diced celery

1/4 to 1/2 cup minced onion

1/4 cup dried cranberries (or more to taste)

2 teaspoons ground curry

4 teaspoons olive oil

1 tablespoon vinegar (white balsamic or apple cider)

1/2 teaspoon kosher or sea salt to taste

1/8 teaspoon freshly ground black pepper

Nutritional Breakdown

For 1/6 of this recipe (about 2/3 cup):

Protein 6.5 g, Fiber 6 g, Sodium 29 mg, Total fat 1.2 g, Saturated fat 0g, Total carbs 31 g, Sugars 5.8 g, Calories 169 Kcal

Directions

Preheat oven to 400°F.

Place the farro in a medium saucepan covered with about 2 cups of water; bring to a boil. Cover, reduce heat to medium low, and cook fifteen minutes, or until tender. Drain excess water.

Toss butternut squash with 2 teaspoons of the olive oil, 1/2 teaspoon of the coriander, and some salt; roast in the oven until tender and browned, about fifteen minutes. For a more charred squash, turn the broiler to brown up the edges, but be careful not to burn them (optional).

Add 1 teaspoon of the oil to a skillet and heat over medium heat. Place the minced onion in the skillet and cook until translucent. Add the celery and cook for a minute or two longer. Combine the curry, 1 teaspoon of the oil, vinegar, 1 teaspoon of cumin, cooked farro, cranberries, salt, and pepper with the onions and celery. Cook for a minute or two while mixing the ingredients together. Toss the kale and roasted squash into the mixture, cover, and turn off the heat for a few minutes so the steam softens the kale. Serve. Refrigerate leftovers.

Mango Quinoa Black Bean Salad

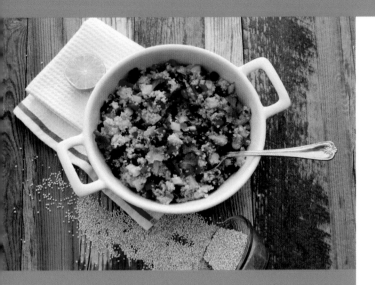

I went to visit my brother, Bill Scharman, and I found him cooking up a storm. He was using many of the "healthy challenge" ingredients from my website, www.foodswithjudes.com, and he had created this delicious salad. It's wonderful and is packed with healthy nutrients. Quinoa, a complete protein, combined with crunchy celery, sweet tangy mango, and lime, makes this salad a winner.

Ingredients

2 1/2 cups quinoa, cooked (3/4 cup dry)

1 cup celery, chopped small

1 red bell pepper, diced

3 green onions, diced

1 firm mango, diced

1/4 cup cilantro (to taste)

1 can black beans, drained and rinsed

Dressing:

2 tablespoon olive oil

4 tablespoons red wine vinegar

2 tablespoon lime juice

2 tablespoon raw honey or real maple syrup

salt and pepper to taste

Nutritional Breakdown

For 1/8 of this recipe (about 2/3 cup):

Protein 3.3 g, Fiber 3.6 g, Sodium 13 mg, Total fat 5.4 g, Saturated fat 0.8 g, Total carbs 19.6 g, Sugars 9.3 g, Calories 137 Kcal

Directions

Cook quinoa with 1 1/2 cups water as directed by the package. Meanwhile, chop the celery, red pepper, onions, and cilantro. Mix these ingredients with the black beans in a bowl. Add the cooled quinoa (my brother throws the cooked quinoa, pan and all, in the freezer while he finishes the other ingredients) and toss.

Mix the olive oil, red wine vinegar, lime juice, and raw honey together to make the dressing. Add the dressing to the salad and serve. If serving the salad later, set aside some of the dressing to add to the salad just prior to serving, and keep the salad in refrigerator to chill.

Chapter 5: Time Your Food

 Visit FoodsWithJudes.com/book-content for recipes, articles and videos.

Seaweed Snack Attack

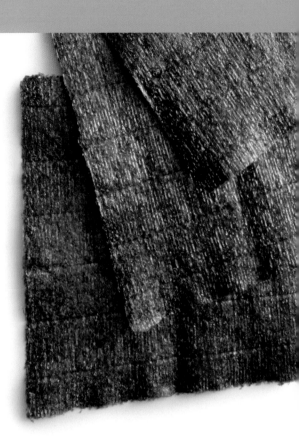

Many of the people I work with say their jobs and families keep them in constant motion, it's a challenge for them to find the time to eat healthy—especially when they just need something quick at their desks or on the go. I offer a series of classes to my corporate clients, and one of them is my Snack Attack nutrition class that lets people actually experience fit, quick snacks for themselves.

For this class, I show up at a business with a mystery bag of food. My participants usually sit at tables facing me. "All right," I say, "how many of you believe that healthy snacks can be just as quick as anything that comes out of a vending machine?"

Then I start pulling out snack after snack: frozen mangoes, apples dipped in lime juice, almonds, lime or peanut butter popcorn, pistachios in their shells, frozen mousse bananas. Volunteers pass out samples to the class. People taste them, have fun, and really get into it.

That's when I pull out the seaweed snacks.

"These are one of my standards," I say, holding up the packets of thin, square sheets. "Now I have to say, the texture is a little weird—like a piece of paper. But they are delicious!

Then someone always blurts out, "No."

"Just taste it," I say. "You might be surprised."

Most of them taste it. They twist their faces up as they're putting it in their mouths. Then all of a sudden, their eyes go wide. "Oh! This is actually good!" they announce. And the whole class starts to talk. "Where do you get those? They really are delicious!"

I tell them which regular stores they can find them in, such as Costco and Trader Joe's, and I remind them that there's no prep involved with seaweed snacks. They literally take no more time to pick up than a bag of potato chips.

After one of these classes, a corporate head came up to me. "You know, we had a lot of classes. Why is it that so many people came to your nutrition class?"

"Well, where there's food, there are people," I told her.

Time to Eat

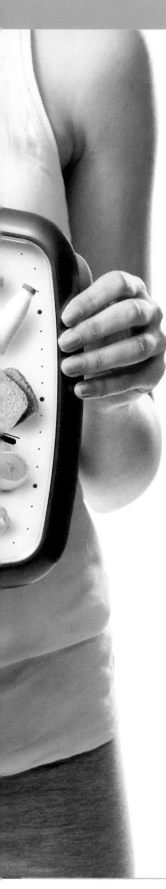

Timing can change the game when it comes to nutritious eating. Both when you eat and the time it takes to eat healthy food can make or break your weight loss attempts.

To lose fat weight, build muscle most efficiently, and keep our brains focused, we need to eat certain types of foods at certain times of the day. It's easier to do than it sounds. I have a few simple, general rules of thumb that you can follow.

66

To lose fat weight, build muscle most efficiently, and keep our brains focused, we need to eat certain types of foods at certain times of the day.

99

There are going to be times when you can't follow my timing suggestions. If you adopt an early dinner routine, for instance, but your friends invite you to a late dinner one night, that's okay. Making an exception once in a while isn't a problem. Keep your focus on the positive. The more often you avoid eating after seven or eight o'clock at night, the better. The goal is to follow these fixes the majority of the time for the rest of your life, not just as a short term commitment.

Timing your food falls into two major categories: eating at the right time of day, and finding healthy choices when there isn't much time to eat.

Eat on Time

People who eat their calories during the day eat less and weigh less than people who consume those calories later in the evening. You tend to lose more fat weight when you eat during the day— even if you eat exactly the same foods as someone who eats those foods late at night.

Eating during the day gives you more energy. You are fueled to exercise more, think better, and feel better overall. At night, you don't move around as much. Yet that's the time when it's tempting to eat foods that aren't good for you: high-fat, sugary, processed snacks.

Your movement during the day helps you build muscle if you are eating enough protein over the course of the day, as I mentioned in Chapter 4. The essential amino acids we break down from the protein we eat may be used up and unavailable to build new protein in just a few hours. To keep enough amino acids available to build and repair muscle, we need to replenish them by pacing our protein intake. In other words, timing your protein can help you magnify your movement so you can build more muscle. This will help you become stronger and healthier and to manage your weight.

When you eat during the day, and especially when you eat a high-protein breakfast, you're less hungry throughout the afternoon and even through the evening. In fact, wholesome breakfast protein makes processed snacks easier to resist.

High-Protein Breakfast

Only half of Americans eat breakfast. Yet breakfast really is the most important meal of the day. Eating breakfast enhances weight loss, improves memory, and boosts performance at work or at school. But that doesn't mean that all breakfasts are created equal.

The best breakfast to sharpen your brain and slim your body is a breakfast rich in healthy protein.

 # Did You Know?

According to Dr. Heather Leidy, Lead Researcher and Assistant Professor in the Department of Nutrition and Exercise Physiology at the University of Missouri, protein-rich breakfasts reduce hunger and keep you satisfied all day long. Breakfast that is chewed rather than drunk suppresses the reward-driven part of the brain, so you're less likely to crave unhealthy, processed snacks in the late afternoon and at night, when your willpower is particularly weak. When you eat a high-protein breakfast, you increase your nutrient intake and lower your calorie intake through the day. That makes it easier to lose weight!

Both Dr. Heather Leidy and Dr. Stuart Phillips, and Director of Nutrition, Exercise, and Health Research at McMaster University in Ontario, Canada, agree that a breakfast containing at least thirty grams of protein is the best way to achieve fullness and curb food cravings. Brain scans done on participants in Dr. Leidy's many studies have shown that eating more protein in the morning decreases the activity in the reward-driven, pleasure-seeking part of the brain associated with food cravings later in the day and even at night. Even better, Dr. Leidy and her team have found that high-protein breakfasts increase activity in the executive decision-making part of the brain.

Eggs are a great source of breakfast protein. While egg yolks have gotten a bad rap in recent years, studies have shown that they are really the good guys after all. They are full of important nutrients that people tend to lack in their diet such as choline, selenium, B12, and vitamin D. The cholesterol in eggs doesn't negatively affect our health like it was believed to in the past, and eggs contain beneficial omega-3 fatty acids.

Read More About The Protein-Packed Power of Eggs

 Secret Ingredient for the Best Tasting Scrambled Eggs

 Front-Load Your Eating to Burn More Fat

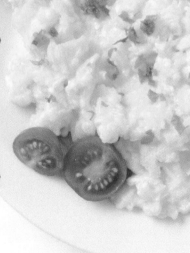

FIX #7

Front-Load Your Eating

You may have heard the popular saying "Eat breakfast like a king, lunch like a prince, and dinner like a pauper." That's actually good advice. Big breakfasts, moderate lunches, and light dinners cooked up with the right types of foods result in more weight loss than do big nighttime meals and snacks.

Boredom, stress, and tiredness can all prompt overeating later in the day and evening. It's not hunger that typically prompts us to eat then; it's our emotions, physical state of awareness, and maybe even our lack of knowledge about the consequences of eating late.

Dr. Satchidananda Panda, associate professor at the Regulatory Biology Laboratory at the Salk Institute in La Jolla, California, found in his research that you burn more stored body fat during the night while you sleep if your body doesn't have as much food to use as fuel late at night.

Try to stop eating after 7:00 p.m. so that you can go about twelve hours without eating. Don't be tempted to just eat breakfast later to space eating between the evening and breakfast for twelve hours. It's important to eat breakfast relatively soon after you wake up to jumpstart your metabolism in the morning. Day, rather than evening, is when you need fuel to be the most productive. With differing work schedules, adjust these concepts to your time frame.

If you have to eat in the evening after a light dinner, choose to eat a small amount of a food higher in protein and lower in carbohydrates, such as nuts. Our bodies readily use carbohydrates for fuel, and the sooner in the evening that they use up the carbohydrates for energy, the sooner they go into fat-burning mode while we're sleeping. When you time most of your eating to happen earlier in the day, you stand a better chance of losing fat weight rather than putting on the pounds.

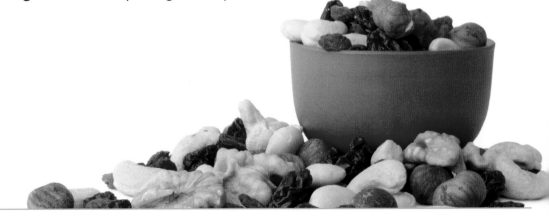

Fix #7 Action Plan:

✓ *Start your day with a high-protein breakfast that you chew rather than drink. If you don't eat enough protein in the morning, you'll be more likely to snack impulsively on high-calorie foods.*

✓ *Don't eat after dinner. Brush your teeth for the night, right after dinner, to avoid the temptation to go snack.*

✓ *Fuel with food during the day to move and concentrate, and avoid food at night when you are not as active.*

✓ *Eat a larger breakfast, a moderate lunch, and a small dinner.*

✓ *Satisfy your food cravings with healthier alternatives such as herbal tea, some raw nuts, or a handful of veggies. This works any time of the day but is especially helpful when you're trying to curb the habit of eating at night.*

✓ *Limit all eating to the kitchen or dining room. Always sit down at the table while eating, and never do other activities (except for talking to people) while eating. This helps curb mindless munching in front of the screen, especially in the evening.*

✓ *Engage in relaxing non-food-related activities after dinner that make you feel better, such as walking the dog, reading, or enjoying a hot bath.*

Track Your Progress on The LEAN BODY, SMART LIFE App

Healthy Foods on the Go

Time is precious. And when it's scarce, it affects what we eat. Think about your go-to snacks and meals. Everyone has them. When you're tired, rushed, and hungry, what do you eat? Do you go out for lunch? Do you rely on the vending machine to get you through the day at work? Do you resort to fast food or quick alternatives such as boxed macaroni and cheese or a pizza delivery for dinner?

When you're on the go and in a hurry, it's hard to resist grabbing prepackaged foods on the way out the door or while you are out. That's why having a few easy snack ideas already on hand or with you is essential to getting you through those hectic times.

Your snacks are a great opportunity to bring more fruits, vegetables, and protein into your diet. If you snack on real food in whole form, it can do wonders for your health. On the other hand, if your snacks are processed carbohydrates, they will be broken down and digested quickly, leaving you with a big rush of insulin, making you hungry again sooner, and putting your body in fat-making mode. To add insult to injury, you are more likely to crave more processed junk.

Even when you're short on time, get in the habit of eating healthy snacks!

There are plenty of natural, delicious foods that fit into any schedule. Make a point to have at least one of them with you at all times, even on a business trip. Nuts, nut butters, fruit, raw vegetables, hummus, and Greek yogurt are just a few of the healthy things you can grab and go. Chapter 3 has several fast-action and fit snack suggestions to use. Remember to always try to include a protein and a vegetable or fruit in your snacks. Arm yourself with great-tasting, healthy snacks at work, on the road, and at home to avoid unhealthy temptations. This is one healthy habit in particular that makes a big difference in your body over time.

The same advice goes for meals. Have three healthy go-to meals as backups off the top of your head. Pick them out as you go through Chapter 8. These meal ideas can just be healthier versions of your current regular default meals. If quesadillas are your backup meal now, change the flour tortillas to a soft corn tortillas and add black beans, a little sharp cheddar, salsa, and avocado, for instance.

It's crucial that you choose your go-to meals in advance to be prepared when you need them. Store the nonperishable ingredients on hand. Keep the perishable items on your mind (better yet, in your smartphone) so you know exactly which items to purchase when you are hurrying into the grocery store, tired and rushed.

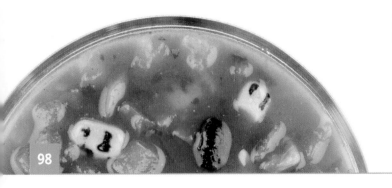

Use weekend or lower-key days to make a large pot of some delicious healthful recipe so there are leftovers in the refrigerator for lunches and frenzied evenings. Use these days each week to wash lettuce and cut up vegetables for meals and snacks. Plan out the meals for the week in advance, make extra food, and prepare for those unexpected chaotic days that leave you either tired or short on time.

 Grab & Go 30g Protein Breakfast

The Seven Most Important Timing Issues for Your Health

As you've seen in this chapter, timing plays a big role in supporting your optimal level of health.

Keep these top seven timing issues in mind as you make small changes for big results:

1. Spread your protein out through the day to help build muscle and to feel full longer.

2. Eat 30 to 40 grams of protein at breakfast to lose fat weight and avoid food cravings.

3. Front-load your calories. Stop eating as soon after 7:00 pm at night as possible.

4. Prepare healthy snacks in advance to eat on the run and have in reach at the office or home.

5. Determine three quick health-promoting meals that you can depend on for easy backup meals.

6. Slow down your eating by cutting each bite in half and by chewing each bite slowly and completely.

7. Eat only when you're hungry, and stop eating when you're barely full.

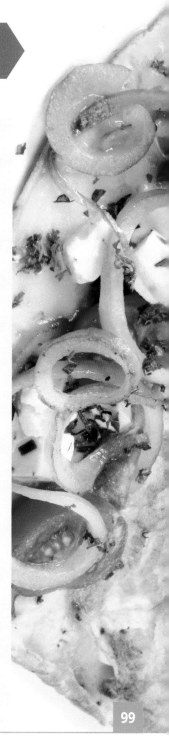

The Hunger Pangs

Learning to get in touch with your hunger signals is essential for getting you to a healthy weight—and keeping you there. All of us can tell when we are hungry and full. We just need to relearn how to listen to our bodies, the way we did when we were babies and toddlers.

By the time we are about three years old, we start to ignore our bodies' hunger signals. Americans are conditioned by our culture to eat regardless of whether we are actually hungry. Most of us grew up with TV commercials promoting processed foods, were encouraged to eat super-sized portions from restaurants, and listened to well-meaning parents telling us to "eat, eat, eat!"

All of those are external cues. A study by Brian Wansink, PhD, Director of the Cornell Food and Brand Lab, found that people who rely on external cues to tell them when to stop eating are heavier than are those who rely on internal cues.

Wansink interviewed 133 participants from Paris and 145 participants from Chicago. When Wansink asked them, "How do you know when you are through eating dinner?" he received two distinctly different responses. The Parisians said they knew when they were done with a meal "when I feel full or when the food no longer tastes good." Chicagoans answered that they were done with a meal "when everyone else (at the table) is done or when my plate is empty."

The participants of Parisian group was leaner than the American group.

That's not a coincidence!

Look at your eating patterns. Do you tend to focus on a computer or TV screen while eating rather than on when your body is full? Do you tend to eat a snack at 2:00 in the afternoon—even when you're not hungry? When you really think about it, you may find that you eat when you "feel" like it instead of when you're truly hungry.

How you respond to eating cues can have a big impact on your weight. If you want to avoid overeating, pay more attention to what your body is telling you rather than to what is left on your plate! When you train your brain to eat based on your body signals, you prevent weight gain and digestive issues. Plus, it feels great to be in control of your body instead of letting external signals control your eating—and consequently your health.

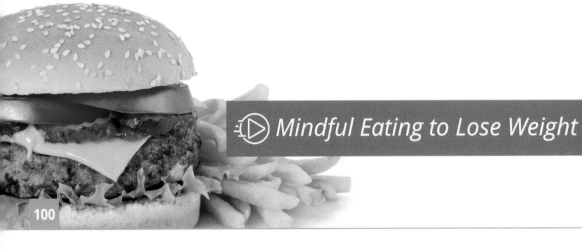

Mindful Eating to Lose Weight

FIX #8

Chew Small Bites of Food Slowly and Completely, Eat Only When You're Hungry, and Stop Eating Just Before You Get Full

To maintain a healthy weight throughout your life, you need to regulate the amount of food you eat by how hungry you are—not by the amount of food within your reach.

Chewing slowly gives your brain more time to realize that you're full. You've probably heard that before, but I bet you don't realize how hard it is to do or how powerful. Try to chew your food until there's nothing left to chew anymore. You will be surprised at the large chunks of food that slip down your throat even when you eat slowly. We're conditioned to swallow food without chewing it very much.

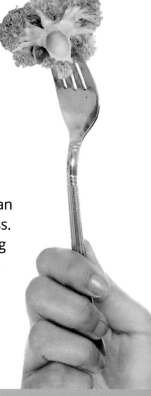

Chewing our food for a longer time tricks our minds into thinking we're eating more than we're actually eating. If you think you're eating more, you actually end up eating less. Ironically, even though we consume less food, research shows that more chomping makes us more satisfied with the meal. Speed eating beats the body's "full" signals to the punch, so we eat more food before the hormones that let us know we are full can peak. Chewing buys time for your brain to tune in and for digestive juices to secrete, making it easier for your body to digest your food, which leads to the absorption of more nutrients and better digestion.

 ## Did You Know?

In a study reported by the American Journal of Nutrition, participants who chewed each bite of their food forty times ate 12 percent fewer calories than did those who chewed their food only fifteen times per bite. That might not seem like a lot, but 10 to 12 percent fewer calories consumed over a few years may translate into a pant size. Practice mindful eating, and take your time chewing as you take in your food!

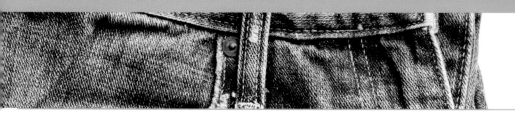

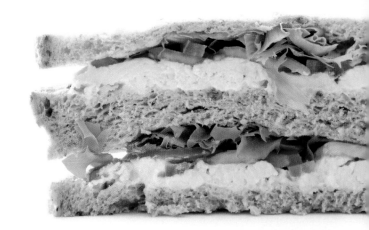

Don't revert to the old "eat everything on your plate" adage. Stop eating when your body starts to feel full. Use the following Hunger Scale to judge how hungry or full you feel:

Hunger Scale

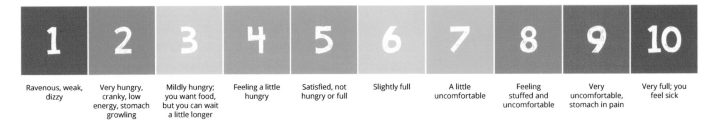

1	2	3	4	5	6	7	8	9	10
Ravenous, weak, dizzy	Very hungry, cranky, low energy, stomach growling	Mildly hungry; you want food, but you can wait a little longer	Feeling a little hungry	Satisfied, not hungry or full	Slightly full	A little uncomfortable	Feeling stuffed and uncomfortable	Very uncomfortable, stomach in pain	Very full; you feel sick

Use the Hunger Scale to help identify how your body is directing your eating. When your hunger is at a 3 or a 4, eat something. Don't wait until you're feeling at a 1 or a 2. If you let yourself get too hungry, you risk overeating. Then, stop eating when you reach 5 or 6 on the scale. Identify what "satisfied" or "slightly full" feels like for you.

Stop using external cues—such as the time of day and the amount of food on your plate—to decide when and how much you eat. Instead, listen to your body's internal cues to determine when you're actually hungry. Keep in mind, you can eat the remaining food later when you are actually hungry. It tastes better when you are hungrier anyway! Using your internal cues to dictate the amount of food you eat, coupled with eating the right types of foods, can help you live a far healthier life.

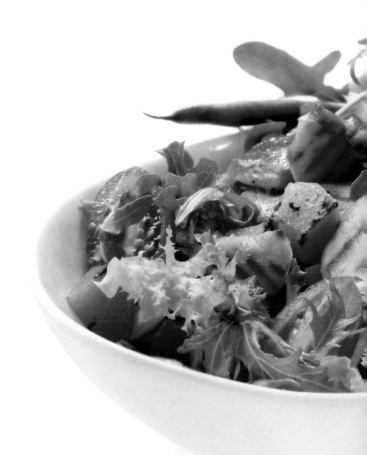

Fix #8 Action Plan:

✓ *Chew your food mindfully and slowly, for longer amounts of time. Avoid doing anything while eating except socializing. Mindful eating means paying attention to each morsel, not looking at your screen.*

✓ *Chew until your food is liquefied before you swallow.*

✓ *Put your utensils down between every bite. Sip water between bites.*

✓ *Eat only when you're hungry—that's a 3 or 4 on the Hunger Scale.*

✓ *When you sit down to a meal, stop and think about how hungry you are. If you're not that hungry, make a conscious effort to eat less than usual.*

✓ *Relax before you start eating and enjoy every morsel.*

✓ *Stop a quarter of the way through your meal and check your hunger level. If you're still hungry, keep eating, but stop if you're not. No matter what your parents taught you, you don't have to clean your plate.*

✓ *Stop eating when you reach a 5 or 6 on the Hunger Scale. Get in touch with what "satisfied" or "slightly full" feels like for you.*

Track Your Progress on The LEAN BODY, SMART LIFE App

Protein-Packed Fruit Bowl

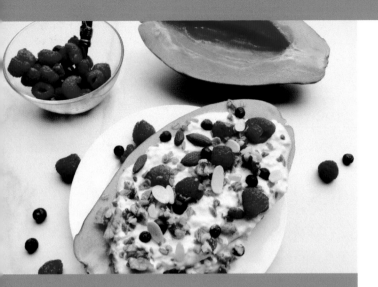

Directions

Mix cottage cheese, yogurt, and maple syrup together. Place mixture in seeded papaya halves, melon halves, or any cut-up fruit of choice. Top with granola, berries, and nuts.

Greek yogurt laced with cottage cheese packs in the protein for the perfect high-protein breakfast. A high-protein breakfast is key to deactivating the brain's pleasure center and helps keep food cravings from taking over, even into the evening. This Protein-Packed Fruit Bowl is a quick, delicious breakfast with thirty grams of protein that is sure to dazzle and satisfy.

If no papaya is available, serve it in a melon half or over (or under) any fruit. Simply mix plain Greek yogurt with cottage cheese and drizzle with real maple syrup or raw honey. In a hurry? You can even mix cottage cheese into a small container of lightly sweetened yogurt and be on your way. No worries if cottage cheese isn't your favorite! The cottage cheese only enhances the creaminess, and the texture isn't noticeable. Don't believe me? Try it!

Ingredients

1/2 cup cottage cheese

1 cup plain Greek yogurt

1–3 tablespoons real maple syrup or raw honey

1 papaya, cut in half and seeded, seeded melon half, or any other fruit

4 tablespoons granola (see recipe in chapter 9) (optional)

1/4 cup berries

1/4 cup nuts

Nutritional Breakdown

For half of this recipe:

Protein 30 g, Fiber 4 g, Sodium 186 mg, Total fat 9.3 g, Saturated fat 1.4 g, Total carbs 31 g, Sugars 14.7 g, Calories 298 Kcal

Protein-Packed Scrambled Eggs

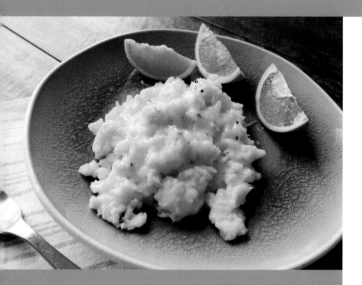

Directions

Prepare a small frying pan with nonstick spray, and put the heat on medium. Whisk the eggs and cottage cheese together until well mixed. Pour into a hot pan over medium heat and sprinkle with the cheese, salt, and pepper. Using a wooden spoon, stir while cooking until done. Makes one serving.

I was surprised that these eggs were so light, fluffy, and good! I hadn't thought of adding cottage cheese to scrambled eggs until I was trying to boost my morning protein. You can use a blender to mix the ingredients, but honestly, no one can tell there is cottage cheese in the eggs even without the blender, so I don't bother.

Ingredients

2 eggs

1/4 cup cottage cheese

2 tablespoons extra sharp or sharp cheddar cheese, grated

salt and pepper to taste

Nutritional Breakdown

For 1 recipe:

Protein 23.1 g, Fiber 0 g, Sodium 405 mg, Total fat 15.7 g, Saturated fat 6.8 g, Total carbs 2.8 g, Sugars 2.8 g, Calories 243 Kcal

Chapter 6: Burn Your Food

 Visit FoodsWithJudes.com/book-content for recipes, articles and videos.

All Calories Are Not Created Equal

Despite plenty of research to support the idea that different types of calories are processed differently by the body, most people still view total calories as the best determining factor to lose weight.

We Can't Seem to Let Go of Our Calorie Levels

Most apps and trackers count calories, perpetuating this distracting calorie-counting confusion. The grocery shelves are full of highly refined carb one-hundred-calorie snack packs, without any regard to their type of calories.

Yet, the 2015 Dietary Guidelines lifted its 30 percent upper limit on fat intake, despite fat's concentration of calories, after four decades of pushing carbohydrates over fat.

Fat does have more than twice the calories of both carbohydrates and protein, so it seems to make sense that eating fat, regardless of the type, would make us fat. It's clear that jumping to that conclusion has gotten us heavier and sicker in the last forty years.

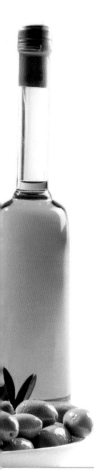

A Mediterranean-style diet, higher in fat (40 percent of calories) than even the typical American diet (34 percent of calories) promotes protection against chronic disease and weight gain. The difference between these two eating patterns lies in the quality of the calories, not the number of calories.

Mediterranean food is rich in olive oil, fruits, vegetables, nuts, beans, Greek yogurt, and fish. Studies indicate that all of these foods help keep fat weight and disease down. The Western dietary pattern, on the other hand, is laden with red and processed meats, sugary drinks, convenience foods made with refined flour, and sweets.

It's true that if you take in fewer calories than you use, you will lose weight. But counting calories tends to be counterproductive. Now, research has given us a better understanding of how sugar and refined carbohydrates, despite being lower in calories, prevent us from burning calories as efficiently and create more body fat. Healthier foods in whole-food form appear to burn up significantly more energy than unhealthy foods; even when they have the same number of calories.

Other factors, like how foods are absorbed and how they affect gut microbiota, also affect how the body treats calories. The utilization of calories is affected by the way calories are broken down, absorbed, and influence our bodies. The nutrients that come along with your calories have a substantial impact on your weight and health.

All calories are not created equal, and losing weight is not just about the total calories eaten. It's about better food burning more efficiently.

Lose Fat, Keep Muscle

Losing fat weight and increasing muscle is a very effective way to decrease debilitating chronic diseases. But for most, it's a challenge to make these lasting weight changes.

Some of it is psychological. We buy into the all-or-nothing dieting mentality that discourages us and eventually breaks our willpower. We get distracted by counting calories instead of focusing on the types of calories. Besides burning less fat with the wrong type of foods, this concentration on calories encourages us to get the total calorie number down lower and lower. Reducing too many calories lowers the number of calories our body burns, which makes it harder to lose weight. Slimming down doesn't have to be so hard!

Not all weight loss is the same. We don't want our bodyweight to be composed of excess fat, but rather of more lean muscle tissue and less fat. The more often we gain and lose weight, the less muscle mass we retain. Interestingly, when you gain weight, most of it is often fat weight if you are not exercising on a regular basis. However, when you lose weight, some of the weight you lose comes from your lean tissue. So over time, if you gain and lose weight repeatedly, your body fat percentage goes up and your lean tissue percentage goes down.

Why Should This Matter To You?

Well, the less lean tissue mass we have, the weaker we are—and the fewer calories we burn even when we aren't moving. At the same time, the more body fat we carry, the more chronic inflammation we have, the more sluggish we feel, and the more medical bills turn up in our mailboxes.

Counting calories is a misdirected battle. We have to redirect our focus to where it really needs to be: on eating healthy foods that make it easier for us to build muscle, burn off extra fat—and keep that fat off.

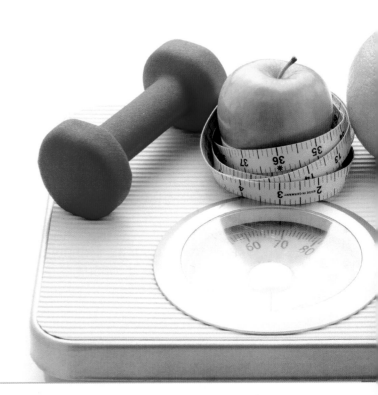

Burn Whole Foods

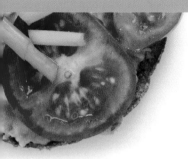

When you concentrate on eating whole, delicious foods, you empower yourself to take your weight—and your health—into your own hands.

Burn More Calories

The thousands of nutrients in whole foods work synergistically to help you burn more fat weight and boost your health. The fiber, protein, fat, and other phytonutrients found in whole foods keep your blood sugars stable and fat ready to burn for energy. Without these nutrients in our diets, carbs break down and rush into the blood too quickly, causing the body to respond with a big influx of insulin.

Too much insulin at once puts your body in fat-storing mode, making it harder to burn off the calories you ate. Those calories are locked up and less available for the body to use as energy. Consequently, there is an increase in hormones that tell you to eat in an attempt to obtain energy.

We want the calories we eat to be used for energy, not stashed in our fat cells. Without insulin rushes directing the fat cells to store calories, our bodies can more fully and efficiently burn calories just eaten to use for energy. Foods in their whole form help you burn fat instead of storing it, and your body takes in many more beneficial nutrients along the way.

By making fruits and vegetables half of every meal and every snack and eating just three whole grain servings every day, you've got your fiber covered and more. A word to the wise; eat fiber naturally in whole foods. Don't be fooled by fiber taken from whole foods and added to high-fiber granola bars or cereal.

Our bodies react differently to different types of calories. Foods from refined carbohydrates such as white flour and sugar slow down our ability to burn calories. They cause our bodies to release more fat-storing insulin and make us hungrier faster craving more refined carbs.

Even ignoring the thousands of nutrients gained from whole foods, studies indicate that whole-grain foods burn more calories than processed foods. It takes energy to digest food. People use about 10 percent of their calories digesting and absorbing food, and eating food closer to mother nature's package seems to take more energy to process.

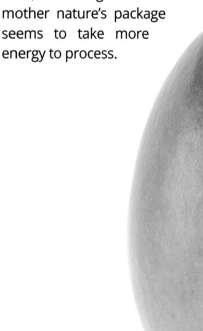

Another study recently published in the American Journal of Clinical Nutrition suggested that eating whole grains instead of refined grains burns more calories and increases metabolism. For the first two weeks of this tightly controlled study, 81 men and women, ages 40 to 65, ate the same foods, including grains, in amounts that maintained their individual weights. For the following six weeks, they ate nearly identical foods at previous calorie levels, except their grains were either whole or refined grains.

Those designated the whole grain foods absorbed fewer calories and burned more calories at rest. In fact, whole grain eaters burned up to 100 more calories per day than those assigned to eat refined grains.

When sugars and starches are stripped of their fiber, the body doesn't have to work as hard to break down and absorb them. And over time, excess calories from processed foods add up fast. Eating whole grains burns more calories, leaving fewer of them to be stored as fat.

Nut and Peanut Phenomenon

Let's talk nuts. Nuts are an excellent example of whole foods that can help you lose weight and boost your health, despite their concentrated source of calories.

The vast results of nut research point to a single conclusion: frequent consumption of nuts leads to better weight control and less heart disease. You may remember the Harvard study I mentioned in Chapter 1 that evaluated little habits contributing to 120,877 participants' weight over a twenty-year period. They reported that the kinds of calories eaten seemed to be more important than the number of calories consumed. Those who lost the most weight were the participants who ate yogurt, nuts, and nut butter.

Many other studies suggest eating nuts and peanuts promote little or no weight gain if consumed frequently, but in moderation. Nuts are loaded with monounsaturated fats which have been shown to decrease abdominal fat. They are also high in fiber and protein, which can keep you feeling full longer. The vitamins, minerals and phytonutrients in nuts and peanuts most likely play a role too.

There are also other factors that contribute to this nut and peanut phenomenon. It takes calories to break down and digest nuts and peanuts, and we absorb fewer calories from minimally processed foods like nuts.

A study from Purdue University evaluated and compared the fat absorption of ingested peanut butter and whole peanuts. All the fat in the peanut butter was absorbed, while only 62 percent of the fat in whole peanuts was absorbed.

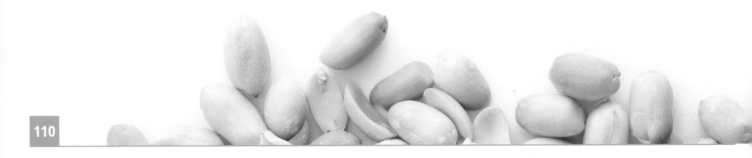

No doubt eating this food in its whole food form allows many mechanisms to work together to promote a healthy body composition and improve your health. In fact, there is even research indicating that those who eat nuts regularly in modest amounts live longer.

Gut microbiota help to break down the food you eat and appear to contribute to the whole food calorie puzzle. They play a major role in digestion, storage, and burning calories in your food. Gut bacteria influences the number of calories absorbed from your diet and may add about 140 to 180 kcal/day to energy absorption.

It appears that low-fiber diets are associated with the microbiome absorbing more calories out of food, leading to significant weight changes over time. Diets with more plant-based starch and dietary fibers instead of animal fat and protein result in more calorie loss in stools, which can be helpful in managing your weight.

It's amazing that gut microbes have so much influence on how many calories you extract from your food. But it's critical to know that food patterns similar to the Mediterranean-style diet (olive oil, fruits, vegetables, nuts, beans, Greek yogurt, and fish) and my 12-FIX LEAN LIFE PLAN have a significant impact on creating a healthy gut community to help burn those calories.

High-Glycemic Versus Low-Glycemic Foods

If you want to burn fat stores faster, choose lower-glycemic foods over higher-glycemic ones.

It's no surprise that high-glycemic foods, such as bread, buns, crackers, white potatoes, sweets, and pasta made from refined white flour, tend to be low in fiber and processed. The glycemic index is a specific measurement from 1 to 100 of the rate at which a particular food's sugar or glucose rushes into the blood. The smaller the number, the less impact the food has on your blood sugar. The sugars found in high-glycemic foods are absorbed very quickly into the bloodstream, and can limit your ability to burn calories effectively.

Dr. David Ludwig, director of the obesity program at Boston Children's Hospital, has been a pioneer in this area. He compared the effects of refined carbohydrates with those of whole grains on both animals and people, and he found that their metabolisms changed depending on what they were eating. Refined grains slowed the metabolism, while whole grains kept it running at a regular rate.

Low-glycemic foods include whole grains, purple potatoes, brown rice, vegetables, and fruit. When we cut back on high-glycemic foods in favor of eating more low-glycemic ones, it changes the insulin response in our bodies. Low-glycemic foods, which tend to be in whole-food form, make it easier to mobilize fat stores to burn for energy.

It's time to rewire the way you think about weight loss. Don't count calories. Concentrate on eating whole foods. Plenty of research makes it clear that highly processed foods undermine our metabolisms. So get excited about experiencing fresh new foods! Don't think about all the things you can't eat. Focus on all the wholesome foods you can enjoy every day. Start appreciating the quality of the food you're putting into your body.

The extreme amounts of sugar and high-fructose corn syrup consumed now is a real problem because the rapid rate of absorption of processed food fructose hits the liver all at once. Our liver isn't designed to handle that much fructose at one time. Eating more than a small amount at one time of high-fructose corn syrup, white or brown sugar (because it's 50 percent fructose), agave nectar (high in fructose), or refined honey at one time can cause the fructose to spill over into the metabolic pathway that leads to fat production. This fat tends to be harmful fat around the middle.

The good news is that the fructose in whole fruit form is absorbed slowly enough that the liver can handle eating plenty of it, even at one time. Fructose, the type of sugar in fruit, isn't inherently bad. Nor is glucose, which is broken down from carbohydrates to provide energy to every cell in the body. The body handles both these sugars well when eaten in whole foods closer to how Mother Nature made them.

On the opposite side, the rapid rate of absorption of fructose and glucose from so much processed food and drink is making us overweight and sick. Drinking calories, even healthy drinks, doesn't allow your body as much opportunity to burn the calories from the food you eat. To burn fat most efficiently, keep your body hydrated, to keep fat cells swollen with water. Drink water at meals instead of beverages containing calories.

Fructose Fallacy

Fructose doesn't spike our blood sugars like glucose can. Consequently, processed sweeteners higher in fructose, like agave nectar, with a lower glycemic index appear to be a healthier choice. But fructose can promote body fat as well. In fact, fructose can cause dangerous fat that surrounds our organs, creating a fatty liver and disease-promoting belly fat.

Realizing it could replace fats with inexpensive refined carbohydrates back in the 1970s, the food industry has had a field day using high-fructose corn syrup in foods. Processed, packaged food became the way, replacing high-fat whole foods such as nuts, avocados, and cheese. Particularly problematic is the amount of high-fructose corn syrup in soda. We've increased our sugar too, which is half fructose and half glucose.

Hydrate to Burn More Fat

Drink Up, Everyone

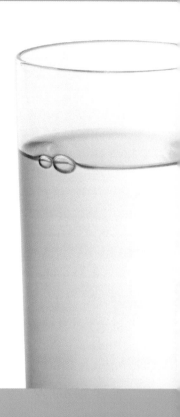

Water can help you lose fat weight and keep it off. Exciting research has shed light on how drinking water helps burn body fat. Cells in our body need to be swollen with water to burn body fat more efficiently. When our cells are low in water, they store more fat instead of using it for energy. Of course, once the cells are completely hydrated, more fat won't be burned by drinking more water. Drinking water all the time ensures that the fat cells can burn to their full capacity.

Drink water instead of caloric beverages during your meals and snacks so that you can burn the calories you are eating more readily. Drinks with calories produce too much insulin too quickly, and linger for too long after the meal. This prevents fat cells from burning as much energy.

Did You Know?

Dr. Jodi Stookey at Children's Hospital in Oakland even recommends replacing milk with yogurt, pointing out that milk was one of the caloric beverages used in the studies revealing water's advantage in weight loss. While diet sodas don't contain calories, they aren't a substitute for water either. The sweet taste of diet drinks may trigger sweetness receptors in the brain to nevertheless stimulate insulin and decrease the breakdown of your fat cells.

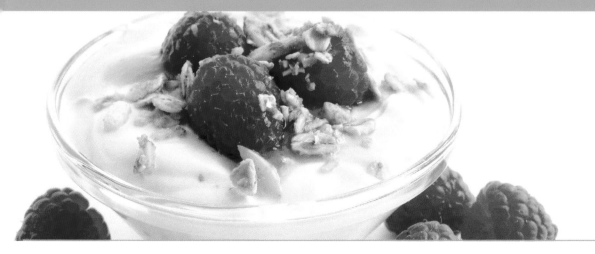

The advantages of water don't stop there. You receive the extra benefit of saving high-glycemic calories when you skip caloric drinks. In fact, research has shown that people don't eat additional food to compensate for calories saved from drinking water instead of caloric beverages (although the same can't be said about diet sodas). Decreasing even three hundred calories every day makes a big difference over time. Given that caloric beverages are mostly simple sugars, avoiding these calories is even more powerful in reducing your fat weight. We often confuse our bodies' signals for thirst as a sign to eat. Sometimes, our mouths just need something to do. Water fills you up, and it doesn't add on calories the way that munching on snacks does.

Drinking water can help us lose weight by revving up our metabolisms. A 2004 study published in the *Journal of Clinical Endocrinology and Metabolism* found evidence that water speeds up the rate at which we burn calories by as much as 30 percent within just thirty minutes of drinking it. That may not sound like a lot of extra calories burned, but it adds up over time, and it is especially significant when water is consumed along with a meal (or before or after a meal).

You've probably heard that about 60 percent of your body is made up of water. Water plays an essential role in digestion, absorption, circulation, the creation of saliva, the transportation of nutrients, and the maintenance of body temperature. Yet the Centers for Disease Control (CDC) estimates that 43 percent of adults drink fewer than four cups of water a day.

When you're low on fluids, your brain triggers thirst, meaning your body is already mildly dehydrated by 1 to 2 percent. Recent science has indicated that your thinking or cognitive abilities can be impaired even at this mild level of dehydration. When we get those cues, we need to listen to them so we can learn, remember, and make better decisions. Water is a nutrient, so think of it as one. Your body loses a lot of water each day through sweat, breathing, urine, and stool. That means we need to replace it for our bodies and our brains.

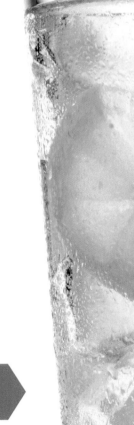

 How Drinking Water Helps Burn Fat

FIX #9

Drink Water Throughout the Day and Evening

Train yourself to hydrate all day long. Keep water ready to drink within arm's reach. Leave a glass of water on your desk or your kitchen counter. Every time you notice it, take a drink. Water fills you up, and it doesn't add calories like food does.

In fact, water can even burn calories if it's cold: an eight-ounce glass of cold water burns about 9 calories more than water at room temperature. Don't be tempted just to drink water and not eat. If you go without food, your metabolism may slow down and offsets the benefits of drinking more water.

To check periodically how you're doing in terms of water intake, take a look at your urine. It should be clear to a very faint yellow color. Douglas Kalman, PhD, RD, a professor of sport nutrition at Florida International University in Miami, recommends you divide your weight in pounds in half to estimate the number of ounces of water you need to drink per day (150 lbs. ÷ 2 = 75 oz. of water). But keep those cells hydrated all the time by drinking water throughout the day rather than at one sitting.

If you're feeling extra motivated, try adding a few drops of high-quality lemon, orange, or lime essential oil to your water. You might find yourself drinking twice as much. Even better, these oils neutralize contaminants in your water and can boost your defenses against illness. Decaffeinated tea, herbal tea, infused water, and flavored water are also good ways to replenish fluids, as long as they don't contain sugar or sugar substitutes.

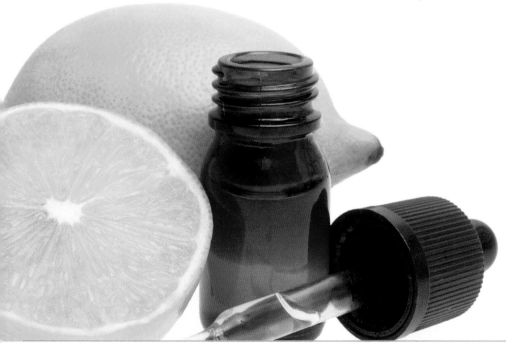

Fix #9 Action Plan:

✓ *Have water with you twenty-four hours a day, seven days a week.*

✓ *Leave a glass of water on your desk and kitchen counter. Every time you notice it, take a drink.*

✓ *Carry a water bottle with you wherever you go, and sip often.*

✓ *Drink water before you exercise, at relevant intervals during exercise routines, and after exercising.*

✓ *Avoid drinking calories in soda, juices, wines, etc.*

✓ *Drink a big glass of water in the morning right when you wake up and right before you go to sleep.*

✓ *Add one or two drops of lemon or lime essential oil to your water. This may offset chemicals in the water and helps to fight toxins in the body.*

✓ *Infuse your water with fruit or herbs for more taste and nutrition.*

Track Your Progress on The LEAN BODY, SMART LIFE App

Burn Protein

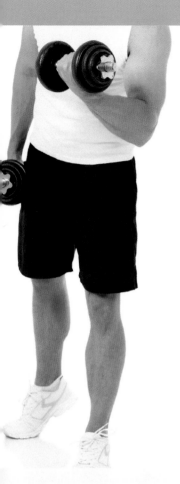

Eating enough protein is a powerful weapon in an attempt to burn body fat and fight against obesity.

There are major advantages of eating protein. Protein has a greater satiety effect than do either carbohydrates or fats, which means that when you eat protein, you stay satisfied for a longer period of time. You become better able to control your appetite, and you eat less. It also takes more energy to digest, absorb, and metabolize protein than it does to process carbohydrates and fats. The more energy you use, the more calories you burn.

Finally, protein helps you to build and maintain muscle mass. Muscle mass is good, compact weight that doesn't take up as much space as fat does while also increasing your strength. Plus, being strong improves your quality of life at any age, but especially as you get older.

The more muscles you have, the more calories you burn—even at rest. Ten pounds of muscle burns fifty calories in a day at rest. Compare that to ten pounds of bulky fat, which burns only twenty calories a day at rest.

 ## Think About It.

You need somewhere between 75 to 150 grams of protein spread out between meals and snacks to preserve and increase muscle mass. The body can use only a certain amount of protein at a time. If you take in more than 50 grams in one sitting, for instance, the extra protein turns into energy (or fat stores), leaving you without extra muscle benefit.

66

The more muscles you have, the more calories you burn-even at rest.

99

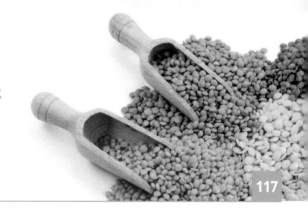

You may have heard that too much protein can harm your kidneys. That's true if you have kidney disease, but this amount of protein is not a problem for healthy kidneys. In fact, 75 to 150 grams of protein is well within the Institute of Medicine's recommended range of 10 to 35 percent of calories from protein.

Studies in the past have not reported problems with this moderate protein amount in diets. Furthermore, a 2016 study from the Journal of the International Society of Sports Nutrition reported no ill effects on the kidney or liver in healthy adults eating double the amount of protein I'm recommending.

Calcium Alert

As you increase your protein, it is important to eat calcium-packed foods to protect your bones. Greek yogurt (20g/cup protein) and cottage cheese (28g/cup protein) are not only packed with lots of protein, leucine (an amino acid that triggers muscle building), and live cultures (which are good for gut health); they are also a whole-food source of calcium. Eating lots of protein without enough calcium (at least 600 mg/day) in your diet can lead to bone loss. However, the combination of protein and calcium strengthens the skeleton and decreases the risk of osteopenia and osteoporosis later in life.

Note: Not all cottage cheese contains live cultures, but are all high in protein and leucine.

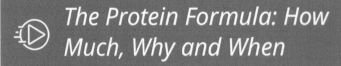 *The Protein Formula: How Much, Why and When*

FIX #10

Eat a Total of 75 to 150 Grams Protein Spread Out Evenly through the Day, with at least 30 Grams of Protein for Breakfast

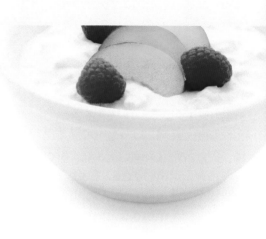

Eat your protein intake fairly evenly over the course of the day to ensure that protein's muscle-building blocks, called amino acids, are always available to build new muscle.

Multiply your current weight in pounds by 0.6, and that will give you an estimated number of grams of protein you need per day to improve body composition: 175 lbs. × 0.6 = 105 grams of protein per day.

To promote more body fat loss while building muscle, multiply by 0.7 instead of 0.6. Also, those in their late sixties or older should multiply their weight by 0.7 to help offset age-related muscle loss. Some athletes may want to use a factor of 0.7 for days filled with extended, intense exercise.

Meals that include nutrient-rich foods from several protein sources are optimal. Protein foods from plants (such as beans, lentils, nuts, seeds, and quinoa), yogurt, kefir, seafood, cottage cheese (the highest source of leucine for muscles), and barnyard eggs are the healthiest high-protein sources. Moreover, they support and satisfy many of the other twelve fixes set out in this 12-FIX LEAN LIFE PLAN. The goal is to make them your primary source of protein foods to contribute to your overall nutrient intake, and to lose body fat, increase muscle, and increase your brainpower, while reducing your risk of chronic disease.

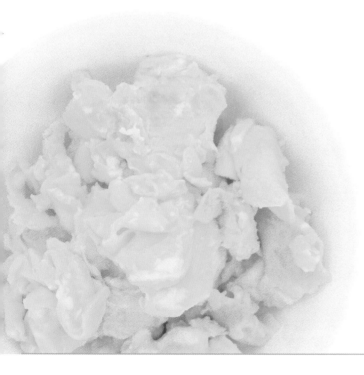

A protein-rich breakfast reduces hunger and keeps you satisfied throughout the day. Studies from the University of Missouri have shown that eating protein in the morning calms down the pleasure-seeking part of the brain associated with food cravings and cocaine addiction. The result? You end up with a lot more control over what you eat—especially late at night, when your resistance to indulgence is at its lowest.

Try to eat at least 30 grams of protein for breakfast and a total of 75 to 150 grams of protein spread out through the day. I've noticed that when I eat closer to 40 grams of protein for breakfast, I'm surprised by how uninterested I am in eating my pleasure foods in the evening. A high-protein breakfast helps you take in more nutrients all day long, giving you more satisfaction with healthier food and fewer cravings for junk foods. This ultimately results in the loss of body fat.

Keep in mind that drinking your protein for breakfast doesn't work the same way that eating it does in terms of satisfaction and food cravings, though protein drinks can help build muscle just as effectively. The lack of chewing causes less satisfaction and doesn't deactivate the pleasure-seeking part of the brain like actually eating protein does.

To get the hang of taking in enough healthy sources of protein at breakfast and throughout the day, track it for a while. Either use the free LEAN BODY, SMART LIFE app or count the amount of protein you eat and write it down. After a few days, you'll be able to recall how much protein these foods contain without looking it up. Remember not to stress out about it. It's better to eat more or less the right amount of protein than to get frustrated and abandon the fix altogether.

For a list of common protein-packed foods, see chart 4.1 in Chapter 4.

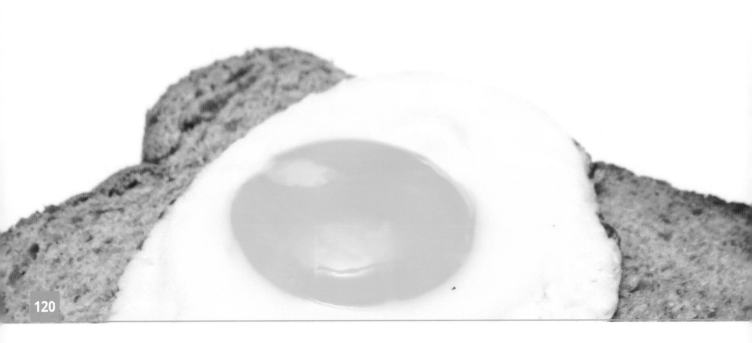

Don't Starve

Because muscle mass burns calories 24/7, it's crucial to safeguard your lean tissue. How? Don't starve—eat!

The protein you eat is critical to building muscle, but it needs to be backed up with carbohydrates from vegetables, fruits, whole grains, and health-promoting fats to protect that muscle. If you aren't taking in enough nutrient-rich calories, protein stops being used to build muscle and is broken down for fuel instead.

Use my 50/50 snack tip and make your between-meal bites half protein and half produce. This snack method helps you eat enough protein spread out through the day to build muscle, but it does more than that. The produce will provide carbohydrates to be used for energy, so all of the protein you eat can be saved to build muscle. All of the amazing nutrients in fruits and vegetables will also help your body in so many ways. Remember, eating fruits and vegetables is your best daily "detox cleanse."

 The 50/50 Health-Boosting Snack Tip

Going hungry often sabotages your lasting weight loss. All-or-nothing dieting encourages drastic calorie reduction without adapting those changes into sustainable lifestyle habits. When you eat fewer calories than you need for basic biological functions, your body throws the brakes on your metabolism and you burn fewer calories. Yikes! The body reacts to these conditions by breaking down precious, calorie-burning muscle tissue for energy. Because muscle is compact and heavier than bulky body fat, the scale may show deceptive results. But losing precious calorie-burning muscle weight won't help you lose fat weight.

When I say "don't starve," that doesn't mean you should feel free to eat a lot of low nutrition foods to get your calories. The calories you take in must be nutrient packed whole foods. Healthy foods that are high in calories—such as nuts and avocados—encourage your body to use fat, not store it. Even better, they allow you to absorb more nutrients, enjoy more food, up your metabolism, and leave your protein free to build and maintain muscle.

Don't go hungry, especially prior to a time when you're more likely to eat unhealthy foods. Always eat nutrient-packed whole foods to help you keep your weight-loss goals on track. I have several corporate clients who make sure that they don't go to business dinners hungry. They will eat a handful of raw almonds and an apple, for example, before they go. It seems counterintuitive, but if they don't eat some whole food before they go, they are less willing to listen to their own bodies' satiety cues throughout the evening.

Fuel for Fitness

I've found that fueling for a game of tennis makes a difference in my energy level on the court. Refined carbs cause my body to drag. I can feel the contrast in my drive and stamina, and so can my opponents!

Nutrition is a critical part of a good workout. You need to give yourself the necessary fuel, hydration, and electrolyte balance to sustain high energy levels and build strength when you're exercising. If your body is an engine, foods are what you use to fill up the tank—not to mention the fluids for the radiator. Without proper fuel and fluid, you're likely to burn out.

There are certain amounts and kinds of protein, carbohydrates, fluids, and electrolytes you can take in to maximize your workouts. These vary depending on the type of activity you're doing, how long you're doing it, and the intensity of the exercise. If you're a competitive athlete, see a registered dietitian nutritionist (RDN) that specializes in sports nutrition for help to become a better competitor. Below are some general guidelines for those participating in less competitive, recreational or exercise-related fitness.

Before Workout

Steer clear of overeating right before you work out. Have an easily digestible carbohydrate snack such as yogurt or an apple to tide you over.Then, eat a full meal within a couple of hours of exercising. Your primary focus before exercising should be on energy and hydration rather than protein intake. Don't worry about eating protein before your workout. The consensus among the leading researchers is that protein intake before a workout doesn't help to increase muscle mass.

Workouts Less Than an Hour

For moderately intense workouts lasting an hour or less, you shouldn't need to eat any extra carbohydrates as long as you eat a whole grain or fruits and vegetables earlier in the day. For morning workouts, drink 8 to 10 ounces of water and eat a banana, Greek yogurt, or a piece of whole grain toast before you begin. Then eat your full breakfast when you finish with the workout.

Workouts More Than an Hour

For intense exercise sessions lasting more than an hour, fuel your body with a mixture of whole grains and simple whole food carbohydrates. Protein before a workout is much less important than carbs for energy. A piece of whole grain toast topped with peanut butter and banana slices will do the trick.

Drink water throughout the day of your workout. One or two hours before the workout itself, drink 15 to 20 ounces of water. Fifteen minutes before you begin exercising, drink 8 to 10 ounces of water.

Intense Workouts Lasting Several Hours

For intense workouts lasting several hours, such as marathons or triathlons, you need to load up on carbohydrates. Eat plenty of whole-grain carbohydrates starting a few days before the race or game. Eat a low-fat, low-fiber, low-protein, high-carbohydrate meal three to four hours before the event. Note that I'm giving permission to eat more refined carbs during this time. Eating carbohydrates before intense training increases endurance by about 20 percent. Whole grains just before an event may be too hard to digest while exercising.

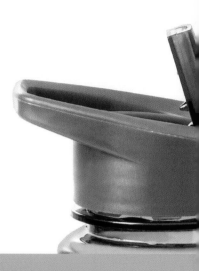

 Did You Know?

Hydration is also critical to be able to think clearly and perform well. Drink plenty of fluids with meals, as well as about 16 ounces of water (5 to 10 mL/kg body weight) two to four hours before the event. Leave enough time to void excess fluids, and make sure your urine is a pale color.

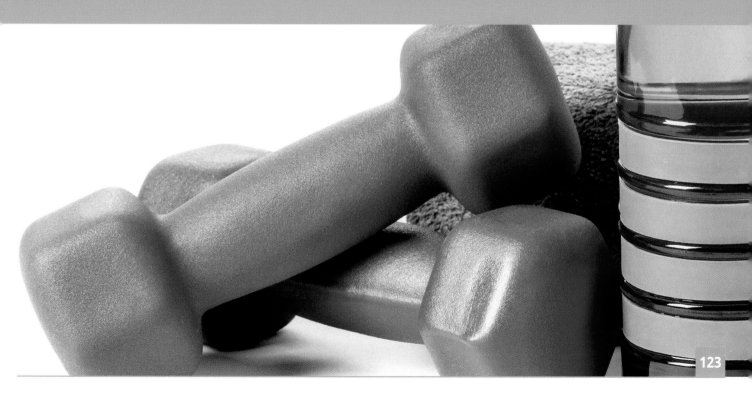

Roasted Potato Kale Salad

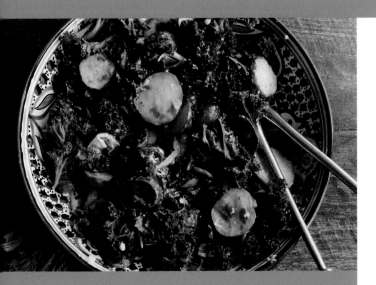

I love this healthy salad! It's delicious and hearty, perfect for the winter. It's slightly warm if you serve it right away, but no problem if you save it for later. In fact, because kale holds up so well, it's wonderful for lunch the next day.

Ingredients

1 lb. purple and red potatoes, scrubbed, cut into 1-inch rounds

1/2 tablespoon olive oil

1/4 teaspoon salt

1/4 teaspoon freshly ground pepper

6 cups kale, stems removed, torn into bite-sized pieces

3 tablespoons red onion, thinly sliced

3 tablespoons blue cheese, crumbled small

1/4 cup sweetened dried cranberries

Dressing:

2 tablespoons extra-virgin olive oil

3 tablespoons cider vinegar

1 teaspoon crushed garlic

1 teaspoon honey

2 teaspoons Dijon mustard

salt and pepper to taste

Directions

Preheat oven to 400°F.

Toss potatoes with 1/2 tablespoon oil, salt, and pepper in a large bowl. Spread them out on a baking sheet in the upper third of the oven. Roast the potatoes, stirring once or twice, until tender and browned, fifteen to twenty minutes.

While the potatoes are cooking, place the kale in a large ceramic salad bowl. Add the red onions to the kale and toss. As soon as the potatoes are finished roasting, place hot potatoes over the prepared kale and cover the bowl with bottom of hot sheet pan ASAP. Let stand for about five minutes while preparing dressing.

Whisk the oil, vinegar, garlic, honey, mustard, salt, and pepper in a small bowl. Uncover the kale-potato mix and add the cranberries and crumbled cheese; toss to combine. Add salad dressing. Serve immediately.

Nutritional Breakdown

For 1/8 of this recipe:

Protein 2.8 g, Fiber 1.5 g, Sodium 157 mg, Total fat 5.5 g, Saturated fat 1.2 g, Total carbs 15.6 g, Sugars 3.5 g, Calories 122 Kcal

Roasted Corn and Black Bean Soup

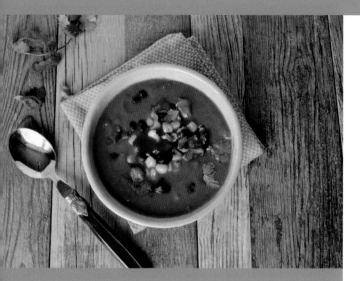

This soup was adapted from Ellie Krieger's Roasted Tomato and Black Bean Soup, but it's a simplified version using canned fire roasted tomatoes and Trader Joe's frozen roasted bell peppers and corn. If you can't find the fire roasted tomatoes in your area or don't have a Trader Joe's store, just roast fresh tomatoes and cut bell peppers along with the onions and use regular frozen corn instead of roasted frozen corn.

Ingredients

1 large onion, cut into large pieces

4 cloves garlic, peeled

1 tablespoon olive oil

1 28-oz. can Fire Roasted Tomatoes or 6 medium tomatoes, quartered

1 1/2 cups or half bag of frozen Fire Roasted Bell Peppers & Onions (Trader Joe's) or 3 bell peppers, seeded and cut into large pieces

4 cups (32 oz.) low-sodium chicken or vegetable stock

1 (15.5-oz.) can black beans (preferably low sodium), drained and rinsed

1 teaspoon ground cumin

1 teaspoon chili powder

1 teaspoon salt

1/2 teaspoon freshly ground black pepper

1/4 teaspoon hot pepper sauce (to taste)

2 cups frozen Fire Roasted Corn (Trader Joe's)

1/4 cup chopped cilantro for garnish (optional)

1/4 cup grated cheddar cheese for garnish (optional)

Nutritional Breakdown

For 1/8 of this recipe:

Protein 4.9 g, Fiber 5.5 g, Sodium 56 mg, Total fat 1.2 g, Saturated fat 0 g, Total carbs 21.8 g, Sugars 1.9 g, Calories 120 Kcal

Directions

Preheat oven to 375°F. Toss the onion and garlic (and tomatoes and bell peppers if using fresh) with the oil in a large bowl, then transfer to a baking sheet. Roast until the garlic cloves have softened and edges of the onions are browned, thirty-five to forty minutes, stirring once after the first twenty minutes.

Transfer the roasted onion and garlic to a blender. Add canned fire roasted tomatoes, frozen roasted peppers, about a cup of the broth, beans, cumin, chili powder, salt, and pepper to the blender. Blend until smooth. Pour the blended mixture and remaining stock into a four-quart saucepan. Bring to a boil, reduce the heat, and simmer for ten minutes. Stir in corn and hot sauce to taste. Heat through and serve with a garnish of cilantro and cheddar cheese.

Chapter 7: Buy Your Food

Visit FoodsWithJudes.com/book-content for recipes, articles and videos.

Supermarket Tours

In 1993, my family and I lived in Boston. I had two little kids, was the author of a supermarket nutrition book, and had a lot on my plate, but I still wanted to help people with their wellness so they could live a richer, happier life.

People were asking me nutrition questions better answered right in the aisle of the store. I thought it would be really useful to walk people through a grocery store and show them exactly what they could buy to eat healthy. So I went to the management of Star Market in Cambridge, Massachusetts and pitched the idea to the management.

Before I knew it, I was running Health-Wise Supermarket Tours in several of the local Star Markets.

Two or three times a week, I walked a group of people through the supermarket, aisle by aisle. We stopped in each section to talk about which foods were healthiest. They asked really interesting questions. I showed them some of my favorite healthy products. While I was at it, I gave them some practical tips about eating good food even when they didn't have much time to cook.

They left the tours feeling happy and relieved to have some new, concrete ideas for fast, fresh, healthy meals and snacks. Back then, people didn't have as much access to nutrition information. Some of them even brought their friends back with them.

It was grocery shopping at its healthiest, and it was fun too.

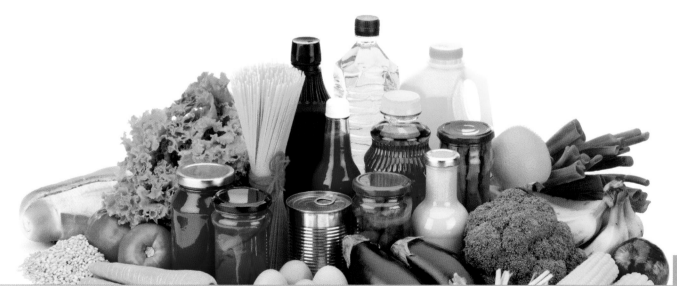

A Shift to Healthy Foods

We go up against a lot of advertising every day that's designed to make us crave unhealthy foods. Fortunately, we still decide what to buy and what to put in our mouths.

More people are shifting to nutritious foods. The more food in whole form you choose to buy and eat, the more you will appreciate the delicious taste of real food. Processed foods filled with refined white flour, sugar, and salt will lose their appeal. You will become more energetic. It takes some willpower not to reach for the bags of chips and cookies on the supermarket shelf during those first few months. But as time goes on, you will start to prefer whole foods to processed foods.

You have the power to change your tastes. And that starts with what you put in your shopping basket.

Produce Convenience

While processed foods in the grocery stores outnumber whole foods, there are plenty of healthy foods that can make your transition to whole-food eating easier and more delicious.

Having a variety of frozen fruit sitting in your freezer all year round comes in handy. Frozen berries pureed in a blender are delicious drizzled over healthier versions of pancakes, waffles, french toast, and plain yogurt. I like to take a handful of frozen blueberries, run them under hot water for just a few seconds, and throw them into oatmeal or yogurt for a delicious breakfast. There's an unending list of ways you can use frozen fruit, and buying it can help you conveniently eat high-nutrient foods.

Produce frozen the same day it's harvested retains its nutrient levels extremely well. Specific phytonutrients called anthocyanins, best known for their deep red and blue colors, need to be preserved so that we can take advantage of their powerful disease-fighting nutrients. Frozen fruit is full of these wonderful phytonutrients along with much more.

Compared to fresh vegetables, I'm not crazy about the texture of many frozen vegetables. Grated vegetables, however, are a different story. Frozen grated vegetables, like cauliflower and broccoli, are showing up in droves in the frozen sections of grocery stores. They look and taste similar to rice and can be used to replace rice in recipes. These riced vegetables cook in minutes and taste great alone, or as a side to your meal. They may be labeled riced, crumbles, pearls or just what they are: grated vegetables that look similar to rice.

While it's easy to make these grated veggies yourself in a food processor, it's smart to have some stocked in your freezer when time or cauliflower are not on your side. As long as these products are just frozen grated vegetables, and no other ingredients are added, they make a convenient way of getting more veggies in your diet.

Buying fresh vegetables already washed and cut means it takes fewer steps to get them onto the table.

Eat Smart sells fresh vegetables that are cleaned, trimmed, and sealed in a stay-fresh package. They offer an array of vegetables and salad mixes with a variety of produce you may never try on your own. A tasty pre-made salad can make your transition from processed foods to whole foods a breeze.

Learn More About Eat Smart Vegetables

Beans, Lentils, Dry Peas

Beans, lentils, and dried peas, referred to as pulses, provide an amazing boost to your health. No other food group can claim to be from both the vegetable and the protein group. Check the labels – as long as nothing else is added except some salt or spices, go ahead and buy these plant-based proteins either dried, canned, or already cooked (produce section) in your stores or farmers markets. I get the best deals in ethnic stores for these legumes in their dry form. I describe how to cook beans easily in a slow cooker in Chapter 8.

I enjoy snacking on roasted chickpeas. My favorite are Biena Chickpea Snacks. They use US Grade 1 chickpeas, with less oil closer to the end of the roasting process for a nice crunch. The texture is crunchy but not too hard like some of the other brands. Sometimes a girl just needs a good crunch, and I'm all about eating my vegetables and protein in one snack.

Learn More About Biena Chickpea Snacks

Organic

Organic foods are great because, let's face it, it's nice to purchase your whole foods without an extra dose of pesticides. A Stanford University study published in the Annals of Internal Medicine reported that eating organic meat and produce reduced the consumer's exposure to antibiotic-resistant bacteria.

The organic movement has generated a lot of hype and attention. "Organic" means that the food has been grown without the use of pesticides, synthetic fertilizers, sewage sludge, irradiation, genetic engineering (GMOs), growth hormones, antibiotics, or other drugs. Also, the food products have been made without food additives such as preservatives, artificial sweeteners, colorings, flavorings, and monosodium glutamate.

To be labeled "organic," products must be organically grown or made from at least 95 percent organic ingredients and 100 percent from non-GMOs. Products that contain at least 70 percent organic ingredients can say "made with organic ingredients" on the label. These requirements are good, but they're not always the whole story. ***Just because something is labeled "organic" doesn't mean that it isn't processed.***

One example is white flour. White flour is wheat flour from which the bran and the nutritious germ of the grain have been removed. That means that white flour is processed, regardless of whether it was grown without using pesticides.

I encourage you to buy organic whenever you can. Just don't assume that because something is organic, it must be nutritious. Processed foods are unhealthy regardless of whether their ingredients were grown with pesticides!

If you can't afford to buy organic fruits and vegetables, don't panic. The same 2012 Stanford study also pointed out that organic foods themselves might not be significantly more nutritious than conventional foods. It's still better to trade in the processed foods for fruits and vegetables. Try buying them in season from local farms for the freshest, least expensive options.

"Natural"

We see the term "natural" on food labels all the time. It sounds good, but be careful. The term "natural" actually has no legal definition in the United States.

Many people assume that if something is labeled "natural," it is minimally processed and doesn't contain manufactured ingredients such as processed sweeteners, lab-produced "natural" flavors and colors, additives, or preservatives. But because there is no labeling standard for this word, it can be legally printed on any food label—regardless of what the package contains.

Be wary of the word "natural" on food labels, and pay close attention to the ingredient lists. If you find phrases such as "added color," "artificial flavors," or "synthetic substances" on the list, the food isn't really natural. Always buy foods in their whole form or products made with whole-food ingredients to truly be eating more naturally.

Genetically Modified Foods (GMOs)

Genetically modified organisms (GMOs) are a controversial topic, and there are definitely two sides to the debate. On one side, the biotech industry and GMO supporters view genetically modified (GM) foods as a way to grow more food and potentially feed millions of starving people, as well as keep rising food prices down. On the other side, many believe that GM foods require more oversight and argue that foods containing genetically modified organisms could potentially be harmful to humans and ecosystems. They push for GMOs to be banned, as they are in Europe, and at the very least be labeled clearly so consumers know whether foods are genetically modified.

GMO supporters claim that Americans have been eating foods containing them for the past fifteen years without credible evidence that people are harmed, yet scientific clinical studies using humans are almost nonexistent. Saying there is no evidence isn't the same as saying GM foods have been shown to be safe. However, when Americans were recently compared with Europeans who do not allow GMOs into their food supply, there wasn't any clear evidence that GM foods are increasing the rates of cancer, obesity, type 2 diabetes, kidney disease, food allergies, celiac disease, gastrointestinal disease, or autism in our country.

Happily, GMO crops have led to a decreased use of insecticides use. Herbicides usage, on the other hand, has increased as genetically modified crops are more resistant to weeds. Encouragingly, efforts to find synthetic pesticides that have high specificity for their targets pests and pest control that is less toxic to people are sure to become part of the permanent solution to this pesticide conundrum.

Surprisingly, the Food and Drug Administration (FDA) doesn't actually require any safety assessment of GMO crops. A limited number of studies have found health issues, including increased inflammation, when animals ingest GM foods.

However, these studies are few compared to the number of animal studies, both experimental and observational, revealing that GM feed is safe and nutritionally on par to non-GMO feed for animals. Given the lack of clinical research of GMOs in humans, the increased use of herbicides, and my preference to eat organically grown foods grown without pesticides, I tend to avoid GM foods.

The majority of corn, soy, canola, and sugar beets grown in the United States is genetically engineered and often used in processed foods and restaurant cooking (mostly due to the oil being used). However, if these foods are organic, you can be assured they do not contain GMOs. The good news is that more and more healthier-type products using corn, soy, and canola, such as popcorn, are labeled GMO-free, and more restaurants are using only non-GMOs. A greater number of non-GM foods will be available as the demand for non-GMOs grows.

Within a few years, consumers will be able to find out whether any food in the stores contains GMO ingredients, because the GMO label law was signed into law July 29, 2016. Food companies will have to reveal whether products contain GMO ingredients, but they won't have to print it on the package label. Instead, you may have to scan a QR code (a type of barcode) with your smartphone to get that information. Small food companies also have the option of providing a phone number or a website URL for more information. While GMO information for foods isn't as accessible as hoped by many, it may be enough to get more companies to avoid GMOs until studies further support their safety.

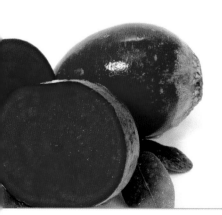

The Big Soy Question

People ask me about soy all the time, but especially when shopping. Rodents react very differently to soy than humans, so the findings that soy causes breast cancer, especially in those that have already beaten breast cancer, have been replaced by human studies that found the opposite was true in humans. So despite a lot of bad press, soy is safe and even beneficial.

The big problem with soy is that it is often over-processed, losing many of its healthy traits. The powerful phytonutrients isoflavones are found in soy foods that aren't highly processed, like edamame. Highly processed soy foods such as soy ice cream, power bars, and hot dogs have much lower amounts of isoflavones.

Many of these products are made with soy isolates. These isolates are formed by isolating the protein from the soybean, and taking out the hundreds of thousands of other nutrients that are meant to work together for your health.

Check your label to see what type of soy is included. Organic products made with soy are from non-GMO soybeans, but that doesn't mean they aren't highly processed. Try eating soy in a whole food form.

Tempeh, natto, and miso are all whole food forms of soybeans that have been made or fermented by nature using good bacteria. That's the kind of soy you want to improve your gut health.

Edamame, a whole food without any processing, is also an excellent choice to take advantage of soy's quality and ample plant-based protein. Fermented and less processed soy is loaded with health-boosting nutrients from vitamins, minerals, fiber, and phytonutrients. This is an excellent way to start moving to a more plant-based diet.

More Information About Soy

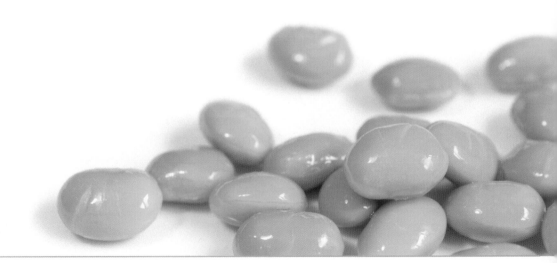

Lessons in Labels

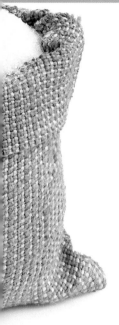

When you're shopping for healthy foods, remember: labels aren't always what they seem.

This goes beyond the claims of "natural" and "organic." Labels are great in theory. In practice, you might be surprised by how many loopholes food manufacturers can find when it comes to making their labels say what they want them to say.

Sugar is a great example. When you look at a label, it gives you the total amount of sugar in the product. What it doesn't specify is how much sugar is naturally found in the food, and how much of it is added after the fact. There is a big difference between the two.

So you have to dig a little deeper. Go down to the ingredient list and see where "sugar" falls on the list. Take a look at what kinds of sugar are included there. Between that and the total amount of sugar in the product, you can get an idea of how much of it is natural and how much of it isn't.

If the sugar were reported in teaspoons instead of grams, it would be easier to see that a twenty-ounce bottle of Coca-Cola with sixty-five grams of sugar has 16 teaspoons of added sugar. There are four grams of sugar in every teaspoon—do the math.

Other improvements with the new labels include serving sizes that better reflect how much consumers actually eat in one sitting. For instance, an ice cream serving will become two-thirds of a cup rather than the current half cup. Calorie counts will be in a larger, bolder font so they will be easier to spot. Most food manufacturers will be required to use the new label by July 2018. Food companies with less than $10 million in annual sales will have another year to comply.

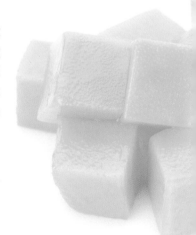

That said, not many whole foods need labels at all. Fruits, vegetables, beans, lentils, whole grains, fish, and nuts are the better bet for your health, whenever you can buy them.

Buy Healthy Eggs

Not all eggs are equally nutritious, and it's important to know how to read egg labels to tell the difference. Phrases such as "cage-free" and "free-range" on egg cartons can be misleading. Just because chickens aren't in cages doesn't mean they're spending time outdoors in a pasture to increase the nutrient levels of the eggs. They're not. They are packed into a room full of chickens without cages. However, free-range hens do have access to a designated outdoor area.

The term "organic" on the label doesn't guarantee that the hens have a natural lifestyle, either. It means only that the hens are uncaged and have some outdoor access, although how much isn't specified. It also means the hens are fed an organic, all-vegetarian diet free of antibiotics and pesticides.

Unfortunately, the term "pasture-raised" has no legal meaning and can be used without regulation.

So how do you identify the best eggs? The healthiest eggs are true barnyard eggs, where a chicken is able to freely roam, eating bugs and worms. However, these are hard to come by. If you can't find a small farm near you where chickens are foraging for food, look for eggs in stores that are "animal welfare approved." This badge means the birds are from a family-run farm with no more than 500 hens and constant outdoor access. That way, you can at least hope you're eating eggs from chickens that have been roaming around and eating as nature intended, thereby boosting the nutrition in their eggs.

The "certified humane" stamp of approval means the chickens have secluded nest boxes instead of cages. Even eggs with an "American Humane certified' stamp on the carton allow the birds to have perches, scratch pads, and nest boxes in their cages. The United Egg Producers approve 80 percent of caged birds, so this certification probably means the birds are treated poorly, resulting in sad hens with less nutritious eggs.

Don't Buy Eggs from Vegetarian-fed Hens

I've noticed that some cage-free eggs are labeled "vegetarian-fed." This term isn't USDA-regulated. But more importantly, you don't want your eggs to be from a hen eating a vegetarian diet. They need to eat bugs and worms, as nature intended, to enhance key nutrients in their egg.

Chickens also need the protein from their foraging finds to consume the amino acid, methionine. Without it, they become ill, because instinctively, they want meat. So when they don't get it, they violently peck at each other in search of the protein they need. So don't buy eggs that are labeled "vegetarian-fed." Chickens are omnivores, after all!

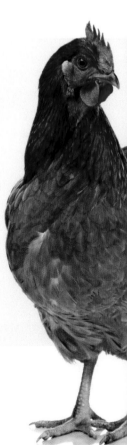

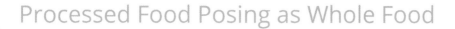

Processed Food Posing as Whole Food

Labels and health slogans can be misleading—especially when it comes to processed foods and convenience snacks. That nutritionally hyped-up granola or power bar you like isn't going to compare to mother nature's real food in whole form.

What they don't tell you is that the makers of processed foods often add overly refined flours, fibers, and proteins to increase the values on their nutrition labels. Those numbers support the superficial claims they make, but they don't often support your health like whole foods do.

For example, many cereal manufacturers are anxious to increase the fiber content of their cereals—but they don't want to alter the original recipe. So they extract fiber from whole grains and add it into the mix. Unfortunately, that fiber isn't nearly as effective without the whole grain itself. In their natural state, the thousands of nutrients work together to create powerful health benefits.

When you're grocery shopping, beware of foods that use extracts of certain nutrients. The longer the ingredient list is on the label, the more probable it is that the manufacturer is using parts of whole foods to substitute for whole foods themselves. Granola and sports bar manufacturers often use this trick to raise the protein and fiber numbers on their nutrition labels. Try to choose brands that pack nutrients into their bars with natural methods, like Kind bars that contain whole-food nuts or whole grains and have only five grams of sugar or less.

If you're used to buying many processed foods, it can be hard to break the habit. Stick with it! After you avoid processed foods for just a couple of months, it gets a lot easier to keep bad shopping choices out of your grocery cart. Your taste buds adjust to eating healthy foods, and the processed foods you used to enjoy are no longer as appealing as they used to be.

Buy Great Grains

When you shop for healthy grains, you need to be familiar with the lingo.

Labels with terms such as "multigrain," "100% wheat," "organic," "pumpernickel," "bran," "wheat flour," and "stone ground" may sound healthy, but technically none of these words and phrases means that the product is actually whole grain.

For example, a label claiming that the product in question is multigrain just means that the product contains more than one type of grain. That can easily mean that it has more than one type of refined grain.

By the same token, "100% wheat bread" means only that the bread is made from wheat flour. That flour may be refined—meaning that it has been stripped of the bran and germ—and the statement would still be true.

When you buy grains, look for the word "whole." "Whole" is the magic word here. Check the ingredient list. If it reads "whole wheat flour" or "whole" whatever type of flour, then you're in good shape. It's best to have whole grain be the first ingredient on the list, meaning that the product contains more whole grain than any other ingredient.

Buy Great Grains

When you shop for healthy grains, you need to be familiar with the lingo.

Labels with terms such as "multigrain," "100% wheat," "organic," "pumpernickel," "bran," "wheat flour," and "stone ground" may sound healthy, but technically none of these words and phrases means that the product is actually whole grain.

For example, a label claiming that the product in question is multigrain just means that the product contains more than one type of grain. That can easily mean that it has more than one type of refined grain.

By the same token, "100% wheat bread" means only that the bread is made from wheat flour. That flour may be refined—meaning that it has been stripped of the bran and germ—and the statement would still be true.

When you buy grains, look for the word "whole." "Whole" is the magic word here. Check the ingredient list. If it reads "whole wheat flour" or "whole" whatever type of flour, then you're in good shape. It's best to have whole grain be the first ingredient on the list, meaning that the product contains more whole grain than any other ingredient.

You might be wondering which breads are the best for you. Ideally, sourdough bread made from a starter full of nutritious microbes, taking three days to make instead of three hours like commercially made bread, is the most nutritious choice. Sourdough made with whole grains and a long fermentation time is the healthiest bread choice. The fermentation process used to make sourdough bread slows down the absorption of the sugar into the blood and is easier to digest. If you find whole grain sourdough bread at a bakery, make sure it's made with a long fermentation time.

Bread that takes three days to make isn't always a viable choice in our modern world. Dave's Killer Bread, sold across the county, offers great tasting whole grain options. I'm particularly fond of the thin sliced varieties, because two slices count as one whole grain serving.

For a healthier alternative for your three to six servings of whole grains per day, choose ancient grains such as farro, sorghum, quinoa, spelt, Kamut, freekeh, millet, amaranth, teff, chia seeds, einkorn, and emmer when possible. They are more widely sold in typical grocery stores now, as well as Whole Foods-type stores, and can often be found in wholesale stores such as Costco for a reasonable price.

I recently discovered a brand of whole grain sorghum that cooks faster and has a nice soft bite, almost like an Israeli couscous, called Wondergrain.

It's naturally gluten-free and can be used like rice. It's in a few grocery store chains on the East Coast such as Select Fresh, The Fresh Market and NE Whole Foods now, but it's growing in popularity, so I imagine it will be available in more places soon. Of course, their website and Amazon also sell it.

Wondergrain

Sprouted Grains and Seeds

You may be wondering about the sprouted grains popping up in grocery stores. When whole grains and seeds are soaked and left to germinate and the new sprout is still shorter than the original grain, then it is considered a sprouted grain.

At this point, there is no regulated standard definition of "sprouted grains," so sprouted products vary. The nutrient changes that occur with sprouting differ greatly depending on the type of seed sprouted. There are also many other variables that go into sprouting grain or seeds that you don't know under what conditions or for how long the sprouting has occurred in these products.

In addition, labels with sprouted grains or seeds may not be a good indicator of how much of the sprouted grain is used. Processed foods may use sprouted grain or seed as a way to lure you into thinking they are healthy. Is the product also made with refined flours? Even ancient grains can be made into refined flour. Look at the ingredient list and evaluate what flours are used and where they are on the list. The higher up on the ingredient list, the more there is of that ingredient. What other ingredients are used, what type, and how far up the list is sugar?

Unfortunately, there are numerous reports that raw sprouts have been linked to more than thirty food-borne illness outbreaks in the last fifteen years. The Food and Drug Administration recommends children, the elderly, pregnant women, and persons with weakened immune systems avoid eating raw sprouts for this reason.

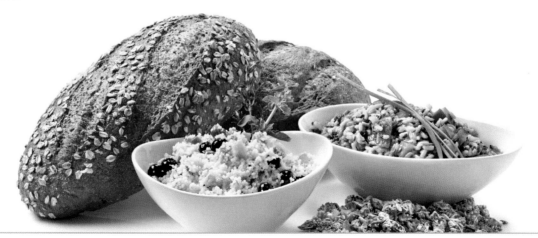

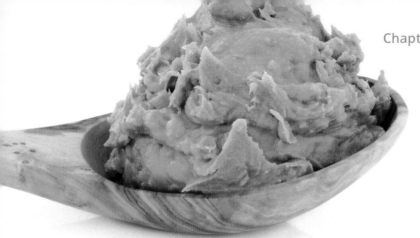

Peanut Butter Stripped Down

I know people want peanut butter sweet and not too oily, but I promise, you will become acclimated. You will like healthier peanut butter if you stick with it for a while. Read the labels. Give brands that don't add extra sugar and fat (especially hydrogenated fat) a chance.

Good old crushed peanuts and salt are all you need to find real joy in peanut butter. Add a little crushed fruit, real maple syrup, or raw honey to sweeten the peanut butter if you want. You will be doing yourself and your kids a big favor, because whatever they get used to is what they'll eat the rest of their lives. If you have a hard time letting go of your favorite added-fat and sugar-laden peanut butter, then you know what I mean. You might as well help them get used to peanut butter that is healthier for them and just as enjoyable (if not more so) in the long run!

Powdered peanut butter seems to be popular but may not be as good of a choice as crushed peanuts and a little salt. The label attracts buyers by boldly displaying that it's "85% less fat calories than traditional peanut butters." As I've said, so many nutrients in whole-food form work together to promote health in ways we don't even understand yet. So pulling out really healthy monounsaturated fat that helps decrease belly fat and then adding sugar to the product probably is not as healthy as regular peanut butter made from peanuts and salt.

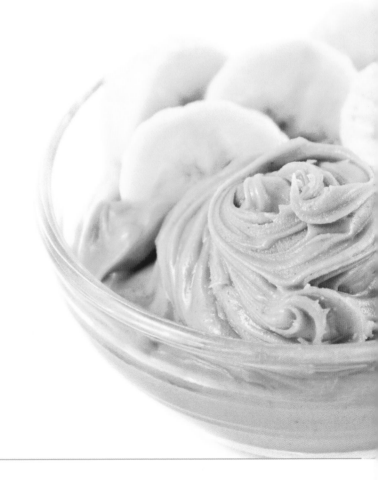

Buying Healthy, Sustainable Fish

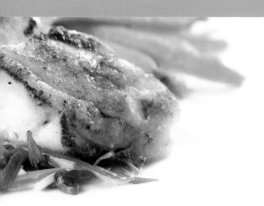

News flash! Mercury toxicity is not an issue in most varieties of seafood, contrary to what was once suspected. Eating fish doesn't cause mercury toxicity; it actually prevents it! The key is the combination of mercury and selenium people ingest, not the amount of mercury alone.

Learn More on Seafood

There is so much selenium in most seafood that it neutralizes the mercury, and you often end up with a surplus of selenium reserves. This is good news, because selenium recycles and restores many vital antioxidants, such as vitamin C, to their active form, protecting against damage in vulnerable tissues such as the brain. Selenium also prevents and reverses oxidative damage throughout the body. All cells need selenium, and there is no substitute for it in the body.

Seafood has other valuable nutrients too, such as active omega-3 fatty acids (DHA and EPA), choline, vitamin D, and iodine, that most people are not eating enough of and that can be difficult to find in other foods. Pregnant women and young children are especially in need of these valuable nutrients but may be unaware of seafood's terrific health benefits. For everyone, eating sustainable marine life is more important to your health than you can imagine, so it's time to get in the habit of buying it.

Americans are eating only 10 to 20 percent of the two to three seafood meals (eight to twelve ounces) recommended per week. People and especially pregnant women have shied away from eating seafood because of mercury warnings.

It's easier to buy seafood now that the mercury toxicity issue is more clear. Just **avoid** tilefish from the Gulf of Mexico, king mackerel, swordfish, and shark (which make up only 0.5 percent of total US fish intake). These are all species of fish that are low in selenium while high in mercury.

Ninety-seven percent of freshwater fish in the United States have proper balances of selenium and mercury, but lake- and river-caught fish are highly dependent on the selenium in the soil surrounding the watershed. ***Be sure to find out if the fish is safe to eat in a particular fresh body of water.***

Purchase seafood (especially wild salmon, anchovies, mussels, rainbow trout, and sardines) that is particularly high in active omega-3 fatty acids (DHA and EPA). These inflammation-fighting fatty acids reduce the risk of cardiovascular disease and stroke as well as many other inflammation-related diseases, plus depression and anxiety. They may even help our minds stay focused.

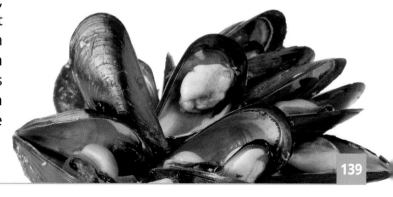

Seafood Sustainability

Catching fish faster than they can reproduce is an urgent issue that is one of the biggest threats to our world's oceans. We want to eat more fish, not less, so we need to protect the fish that we have. Not all seafood is overfished, but we need to be aware of which species are in danger so we don't add to the problem when buying fish at the market or in a restaurant. Avoid bluefin tuna, wild sturgeon, all species of shark, orange roughy, skates and rays, most Chilean sea bass, most Atlantic halibut, and most marlin.

Farmed seafood or aquaculture is another source of confusion and has its issues. Some of these farm-raised fish cause concern with regard to chemicals, disease and parasites, feed sourcing, escapes, and nutrient loading that can have severe environmental consequences if not monitored and carried out in accordance to set standards. However, the growing demand for seafood in the future can be met only through aquaculture. Fortunately, many of these fish farms continue to improve as third-party organizations have emerged and set a higher bar for the farmers. There are now some very sustainably farmed fish available, including salmon. It's important to note that some seafood farming actually helps the marine environment. Oysters and clams, for instance, actually clean the water and keep waters healthier.

Also, branch out and try to choose a different fish variety. This helps build a market for the abundant but underutilized amount of fish, such as scup, that are caught while fishers are seeking other types of seafood. Look for what's local and seasonal if you live near the coast. Take advantage of what's fresh in the marketplace rather than shopping for a specific type of fish.

Healthy, Sustainable Seafood Choices

- Coldwater fish such as Atlantic mackerel, sardines, and herring

- Farmed fish such as US tilapia, US rainbow trout, US catfish, and US striped bass

- Farmed shellfish such as blue mussels, New England clams, US oysters, and US bay scallops

- Wild-caught fish, salmon, barramundi, US bluefish, Dungeness crab, and US mahimahi

Avoid bluefin tuna, wild sturgeon, all species of shark, orange roughy, skates and rays, most Chilean sea bass, most Atlantic halibut, and most marlin.

Also, avoid these high-mercury, low-selenium fish: tilefish from the Gulf of Mexico, king mackerel, swordfish, and shark.

(This information is from the Monterey Bay Aquarium, the Blue Ocean Institute, and the New England Aquarium.)

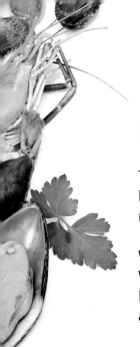

More Seafood Buying Tips

Try to buy fish that is bright and translucent rather than dull. You also want fish that smells like fresh seawater, rather than fish that smells "fishy." It's completely fine and sometimes more convenient to buy frozen, sustainable seafood.

When it comes to salmon, wild salmon from the Pacific, including both Alaska and Washington, is a great choice for the environment and your health. Canned or pouched Pacific Ocean salmon is always available and easy to incorporate into meals, such as salads and main dishes. It's good for you, the fish, and your pocketbook.

I order wild-caught salmon from Vital Choice. Vital Choice's salmon and other types of seafood are immediately flash frozen out on the fishing boat in the Pacific Ocean to lock in nutrients. The perishable items such as salmon fillets are shipped in dry ice and arrive within one to two days. The canned salmon is the best I've ever eaten. It is the same quality as the fillets and has never been frozen like other canned salmon.

Vital Choice

For those of you who are a little iffy about eating fish at all, I recommend trying Barramundi, The Sustainable Seabass. It's a particularly delicious, mild fish that has the highest omega-3s of ANY white fish. You can buy it frozen in stores throughout the country. For stores in your area that carry Australis Barramundi, check out the following website:

The Better Fish

Purchasing seafood doesn't have to be difficult or nerve racking! You need to eat more of it to take advantage of its many health benefits. Use the Seafood Watch app when deciding what seafood to buy. It's so quick that you can find out the best choice while looking over the menu at a restaurant. Fish oil supplements can be a healthy addition to eating fish, but don't use these supplements as a replacement for eating seafood. While fish oil pills are helpful, recent research has indicated the benefits from eating seafood exceed those of supplements. Plus, fish oil supplements provide only active omega-3s without all the many other hard-to-get nutrients found in seafood. Pledge to eat seafood two to three times per week, and start by shopping for seafood today.

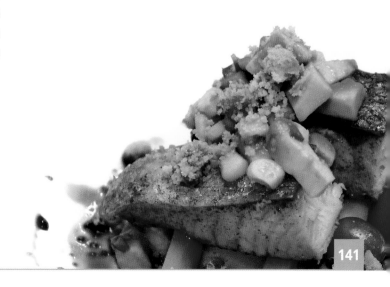

Yogurt Power

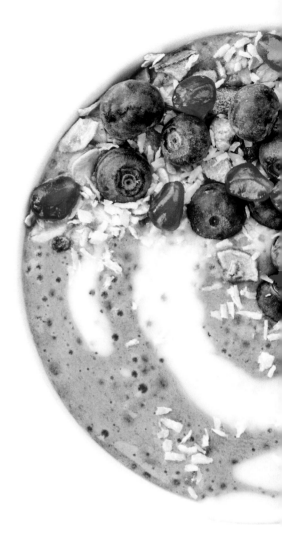

Yogurt is a quick and nutritious food—but only if you buy the right kinds. Greek, Icelandic skyr, and German quark yogurts give you the biggest protein and calcium bang for your health.

Those who don't tolerate dairy well may be having a difficult time digesting the milk, sugar, or lactose found in dairy products. Yogurt is very low in lactose because the microbes eat the lactose during the fermenting process.

Dairy products may also be problematic for people due to what the feed cows are eating these days. Yogurt and kefir made from grass-fed cows or a healthier feed may be worth trying before you give up on dairy foods (especially yogurt, kefir, and cheese) completely. The nutrients and protein dairy offers are hard to beat.

Yogurt can also be completely dairy-free when made with nondairy milks such as soy, almond, rice, or coconut milk. Most of these nondairy yogurts won't provide nearly as much protein or calcium as cow's milk will, but they are fermented foods that can improve your gut flora and be helpful to your health.

Regardless of what ingredients the actual yogurt is made from, many on the market have been corrupted with sugar and artificial ingredients. Follow these seven simple tips to buy the best yogurt for yourself and your family.

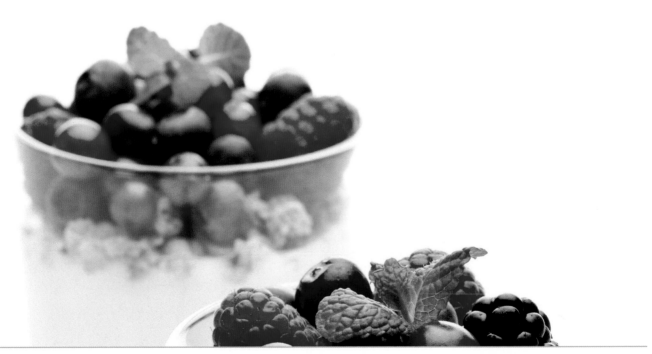

The Yogurt Rules: Seven Tips to Buy Great Yogurt

1. Look for yogurt that contains "live and active cultures." Some companies heat-treat yogurt after culturing it with the good bacteria, killing both the good and the bad bacteria to make it last longer and reduce tartness. These live and active bacteria promote gut health, boost immunity, and may even be a key to becoming slim and trim.

2. Choose yogurt that is low in sugar. Avoid any yogurt that lists sugar as the first ingredient. A standard 5.3-oz. individual container of yogurt should contain no more than sixteen grams of sugar, and ideally fewer than thirteen grams. Shoot for fewer than twenty-five grams of sugar per cup, but fewer than twenty grams of sugar per cup is better. The best option is to add fruit and even a little pure maple syrup to plain yogurt. Another good option is to mix plain yogurt or cottage cheese into sweetened yogurt. This dilutes the sugar and boosts the protein all in one step.

3. Buy yogurt with real fruit. Some so-called "fruit yogurt" is really just a mix of sugar and food coloring. Make sure you see actual fruit on the list of ingredients when you buy fruit yogurt—ideally placed before any added sugars.

4. Avoid artificial sugar substitutes. "Low sugar" varieties of yogurt are often full of artificial sweeteners. If you have to buy a yogurt with an artificial sweetener in it, choose one sweetened with monk fruit. Avoid aspartame and sucralose.

5. Avoid thickeners. Some brands of Greek yogurt cut costs by adding thickeners such as gelatin, cornstarch, gums, lecithin, carboxymethylcellulose, polysorbate-80, and pectin instead of straining the yogurt to make it thick and creamy (which more than doubles the protein and lowers the lactose). These Greek yogurt impostors are often labeled "Greek style." Authentic Greek yogurt doesn't contain these thickening agents or has minimal amounts of them. A good Greek yogurt should have twelve to sixteen grams of protein per 5.3-oz. serving, or nineteen to twenty-three grams of protein per cup.

6. Keep it simple. All you need to make yogurt is milk and live, active bacteria. Plain yogurt should contain nothing more than those two things. Flavored Greek yogurt can have more ingredients, but the list should be short and filled with words you can identify. Especially avoid added hydrogenated fat, artificial sweeteners, or artificial colorings and flavors.

7. Don't assume that "nonfat" means "healthy." "Nonfat" doesn't always mean "low in calories." Many nonfat yogurts have a lot of added sugar. Go for a version that gets most of its sweetness from real fruit. A higher percentage of fat in your yogurt may not be as bad as health experts once thought it was. But because the protein content often goes down when the fat goes up, lower-fat yogurt can be advantageous.

Eat Healthy on a Budget

Many people think that whole foods are more expensive than processed foods are. In fact, the opposite is true. Real foods in their natural forms are often cheaper than processed foods dollar for dollar.

Half a cup of rolled oats, bought in a large bag, is much cheaper than an instant packet of oatmeal. The only difference is that it takes three minutes to cook them in the microwave instead of one. You have full control of the sweetener you add, and there are no artificial flavors or colors.

 3-Minute Old Fashion Oatmeal

The same thing is true of rice. Half a cup of good brown rice (such as brown basmati or jasmine rice) is much cheaper than a prepackaged rice mix such as Rice-A-Roni or Near East. The difference is that a few spices and maybe some bullion are added to the prepackaged options. If you learn which spices make the rice taste good, it takes just seconds to add them yourself.

Beans and lentils are also inexpensive foods with supercharged health benefits. Pulses are the most cost-effective proteins and are eaten as staple foods throughout the world. The cost per serving of dried peas, beans, and lentils in the United States is 10 cents, while beef costs $1.49, pork costs 73 cents, and chicken costs 63 cents. You can find more exotic lentils, such as red, orange, or yellow varieties, at an Indian or Middle Eastern grocery store for much less than at a standard American store (if the latter sells them at all).

Popcorn is another example. Microwave popcorn seems to be America's go-to snack. Plain popcorn kernels are super cheap, and organic popcorn kernels are growing as the demand for non-GMO corn grows. Yet we pay extra money just to have the salt and butter added to them. It is incredibly easy to throw some popcorn kernels into a paper bag and put them in the microwave. Add your own oil and salt to them and you won't just be helping your wallet; you'll be helping your health as well.

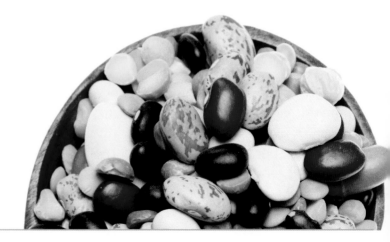

Dinner Ingredients Delivered

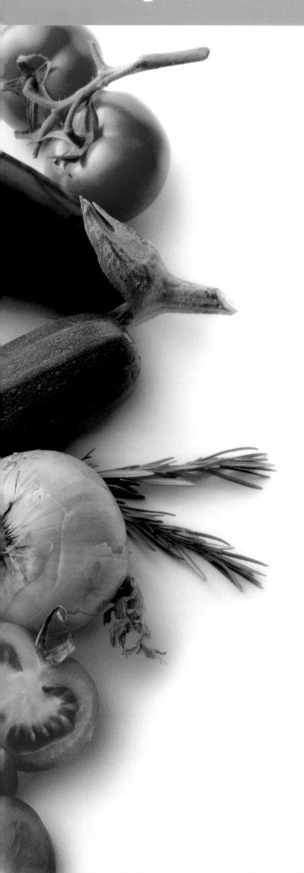

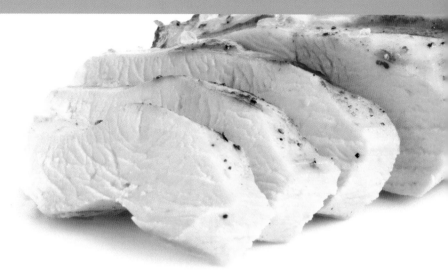

Having ingredients delivered to your door is magical. That's coming from someone who loves to cook. These services certainly make cooking easier and more fun for everyone, but especially for the novice. These ingredient delivery services are popping up right and left. It's another terrific option for your busy life.

There is a cost for the convenience, but most meal kits cost less than what you'd pay in a restaurant for a similar meal. The cost might even be comparable to a meal at home if you are not great at using leftover ingredients, or if you tend to buy fresh ingredients and let them go bad before using them.

These companies are everywhere now. The question is, which services are delicious and healthy? Sun Basket is one that offers delicious, fun food and organic, non-GMO produce, plus sustainable meats and seafood. It also works for most food restrictions. The cost is $11.49/meal, and you are at home enjoying a new, exciting homemade meal in your own kitchen.

Learn More About Sun Basket

Navigating Restaurants

We like to use eating out as an excuse not to eat healthy. We think that if someone else is preparing the food, we're out of luck. The truth is that it's easier than you think to maneuver restaurants in healthy ways.

One corporate client of mine is a champion healthy restaurant eater. Not only does he know how to order, but he has also figured out how to reengineer his environment to help him make good choices. He uses his water glass to block bread, appetizers, and desserts from his line of vision.

If he does order dessert, he often makes it fresh fruit. If he really wants something else, he orders it for the table—that way, he has only a bite or two. Three or four times a week, he will have a glass of wine with dinner, but other than that he sticks to water or seltzer and lime. He figured out early on in his healthy-eating efforts that he just needed a glass filled with a nonalcoholic beverage. He also almost always orders fish—cooked with olive oil rather than butter or cream.

Restaurants don't mind if you ask them not to add butter or cream to your order. You won't always see these ingredients in the description on the menu, but they're almost always in there. Get in the habit of asking for just a little olive oil to stand in for the butter and cream. Drink water until your food comes instead of eating bread. Send the bread (or tortilla chips) away or keep it on the other side of the table and out of sight if possible.

You can also ask for things to be prepared in healthy ways. Fish is a great example. Ask the restaurant to grill it instead of frying it.

Order Salad When You Can

Always request the dressing on the side, preferably oil and vinegar or a vinaigrette instead of a creamy dressing. Instead of pouring your dressing all over your salad, dip your fork into the dressing before you skewer the salad or pour part of the dressing over your salad and mix it up. See how little you can get away with and still enjoy the salad. If you like strong cheese, such as feta, goat, or blue cheese, use it to add flavor so you barely need any dressing at all. Ask your server to hold the croutons and bread.

If an item comes with a side of potatoes, rice, or pasta, seize your opportunity to ask for a double portion of vegetables (made without butter) instead. It's much better to eat double vegetables even with butter than to eat high-glycemic carbs. If that doesn't work, just have a couple of bites of these high-glycemic sides and call it a day. Many restaurants do offer ancient grains or brown rice; a small portion of these healthful carbohydrates can be a great choice too.

When you don't have time for a sit-down restaurant, skip the drive-thru! Fast food is not your only option. Chipotle-style or fast-casual restaurants, from Indian to Mediterranean to Asian to Latin American fusion, are popping up everywhere. They offer us the freedom to choose what goes into our meals and see it happen, all with fresh, quality ingredients. That gives you a lot of control over your order and opportunities to eat more salad, vegetables, lentils, and beans. Don't miss the healthy obsession with grain bowls either. They are a perfect way to eat ancient whole grains with a lot of veggies in delicious, filling ways.

If you're at a Mexican grill, order a burrito bowl. I ask them to make mine with some brown rice, extra black beans, lots of fajita-style fresh vegetables, lots of salsa and pico de gallo, triple the lettuce, and occasionally some grilled chicken or grilled fish if they have it. Not only is it healthy, but I don't usually eat the whole bowl. I save the rest of it for another quick meal later, when I get hungry again.

Even Chick-fil-A offers some quick and healthy options such as grilled chicken nuggets, a fruit cup, and a delicious kale salad. Chick-fil-A also serves oatmeal for breakfast, as do Starbucks and most other coffee places. No matter where you go, be sure to skip the white bread, buns, and rolls altogether. Wheat bread is often highly processed as well but is better than white bread. If possible, skip the bread, buns, and tortillas and concentrate on ancient grains, brown rice, beans, lentils, vegetables, and fruit. Order dressing on the side and eat only some of it.

Don't let the amount of food hinder you, no matter what type of restaurant. Assume you are going to take some of it home for a future meal or snack when you are hungry. You can even split the meal and box it from the get-go. No matter your approach, pay close attention to your body and stop eating before you feel uncomfortable. I promise you will enjoy the food more later, when you are hungry.

FYI, chain restaurants have new menu-labeling guidelines that were initially signed into law in 2010. These new laws took effect on May 5, 2017. Calorie amounts must be displayed for all foods. Just make sure your calories are filled with healthy whole foods that have not been processed. Substitute white rice for whole grains like brown rice or quinoa potatoes and French fries for vegetables, and bread and flour tortillas for lettuce or corn tortillas. Eat fish, beans, lentils, Greek yogurt, and nuts over red meat when possible. Don't pay more attention to the calories than the quality of food, but don't totally disregard them either. Do note how quickly calories from sugar and refined carbs can add up!

Whether you're in a grocery store or a restaurant, healthy food is everywhere. You just have to think outside of the box.

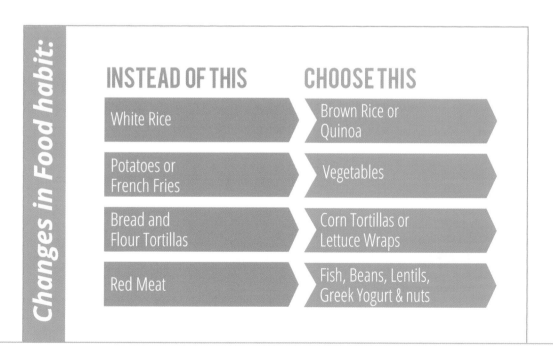

Changes in Food habit:

INSTEAD OF THIS	CHOOSE THIS
White Rice	Brown Rice or Quinoa
Potatoes or French Fries	Vegetables
Bread and Flour Tortillas	Corn Tortillas or Lettuce Wraps
Red Meat	Fish, Beans, Lentils, Greek Yogurt & nuts

Food on the Fly

I fly a lot and I am happy to see an increasing number of healthy options available at airports, as well as trendy eateries offering more nutritious foods. Ready-to-buy packages of fresh vegetables such as celery and carrots seem to be for sale at most US airports. Eat these raw veggies with the hummus that is also available. Even hard-boiled eggs are being sold at many airports in convenience stores.

I've noticed that you can almost always find Greek yogurt, cups of cut fresh fruit, and nuts in these stores, along with salads to go. Go easy on the dressing and toss the croutons. Uncut fresh fruit such as apples and Kind Bars are often found near the register.

The healthiest offering at an airport I've seen lately is an area with lots of healthy options including a salad/food bar in the Newark Liberty and LaGuardia airports. I ate a vegetable omelet for breakfast and a delicious, satisfying, healthy salad full of vegetables, some ancient grains, and protein for lunch while stuck in the airport for six hours. I made good choices by using oil and vinegar rather than the processed dressings typical of a salad bar.

 # Think About It.

If you get on the plane in a starved state, there are often one or two healthier options to buy on the plane. Delta has a fruit, nut, and cheese plate that is full of whole foods other than the crackers. Skip the cookies. These offers change from time to time, but healthy is in, so if you are desperate, it's an option. Just try to stick with real food and skip the packaged food such as crackers, pita chips, potato chips, cookies, pretzels, and bread. Peanuts, even in their dry-roasted, salted form, are the healthiest snack options other than fresh fruit and vegetables because they are in whole-food form.

Bon voyage!

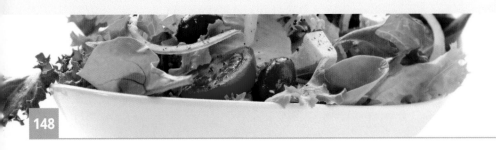
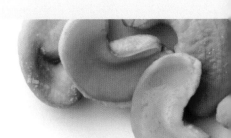

Corner Convenience

Believe it or not, you can actually find healthy options at your corner gas station. These stores are trying harder to sell healthier food and beverages. I recently attended a convenience store conference and was impressed with how store owners are trying to fill their shelves with sparkling water, flavored waters, probiotic drinks, and more 100 percent fruit smoothies. They have more whole-food choices such as Kind Bars, nuts, cheese, Greek yogurt, salmon jerky, fruits, and vegetables.

Even ancient grains are showing their face in this arena. Look for a roasted ancient grain snack called Kracklin' Kamut by Big Sandy Organics that is made from ancient Khorasan wheat called Kamut. The Kamut is roasted, not fried, with safflower oil that is high in monounsaturated fat to help us burn fat, and sea salt. It's crunchy and tasty with 6 grams of protein, 3.4 grams of fiber, and no added sugar per 1.5-oz. serving.

Larger convenience stores even have cut fruit, turkey sandwiches made on wheat bread, and fresh vegetable salads. Keep your eyes open and remember which corner stores offer the healthiest fare. It's going to get better and better given that millennials tend to snack more often.

Kale Quinoa Cheesecake Factory Copycat Salad

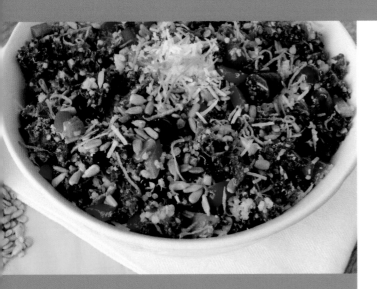

This is my version of a salad from the Cheesecake Factory. I created a version of the restaurant's lemon vinaigrette and added it to some kale, quinoa, grapes, sunflower seeds, and Romano cheese. According to my taste testers, my salad is better! It's easy, delicious, and very nutritious.

Ingredients

1 1/2 cups quinoa, cooked

5 cups kale

1 3/4 cups red seedless grapes, sliced in half (shortcut below)

1/2 cup roasted sunflower seeds, unsalted

1/2 cup grated Romano or Parmesan cheese

Dressing:

2 tablespoons lemon juice

2 tablespoons olive oil

4 teaspoons raw honey or maple syrup

1 teaspoon tahini

1 teaspoon Dijon mustard

1 teaspoon crushed garlic

salt and pepper to taste

Nutritional Breakdown

For 1/12 of this recipe:

Protein 4.1 g, Fiber 1.8 g, Sodium 115 mg, Total fat 8 g, Saturated fat 1.8 g, Total carbs 10.8 g, Sugars 3.4 g, Calories 116 Kcal

Directions

Cook 1/2 cup uncooked quinoa per package directions to make 1 1/2 cups cooked quinoa. Add all the dressing ingredients together in a jar and shake vigorously. Fold the kale in half lengthwise along the stem. Tear the kale leaves off the stem. Stack the leaves on top of each other and thinly chop them. Add the shredded kale to a large bowl. Toss the dressing with the kale and massage the dressing into the kale for a couple of minutes. Add the remaining salad ingredients and combine. Enjoy!

Shortcut: Cut several grapes at once by placing the grapes in one layer on a cutting board. Press a flat lid or plate on top of the grapes. With one hand, press down on the flat lid. With the other hand holding a sharp knife, slice the grapes lengthwise between the lid and cutting board.

Healthy Café Rio–Style Pork Salad

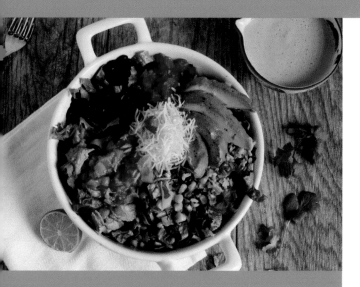

Directions

Place the pork sirloin in a slow cooker and fill the slow cooker half full with water. Cook on low for about seven hours (or for about five hours on high). Drain the water. Cut the roast into thirds. Mix together the salsa, stock, lime juice, adobo sauce (about 4 tablespoons for extra flavor and a little spicy kick), and chipotle peppers to taste if you want the pork to be really spicy. Combine and pour the mixture over the roast. Cook an additional five hours on low or three hours on high. Liquid should cover the roast while it cooks.

Heat the olive oil on low in a medium saucepan. Increase the heat to medium and add the garlic and rice. Sauté for two minutes, stirring frequently. Add the stock/broth, salt, and lime juice and bring to a boil. Cover and cook on low for thirty minutes or until the water is absorbed by the rice. When the rice is done, add the lime zest and chopped cilantro and mix well.

Add lettuce to salad bowl and top with rice, beans, corn, avocado, pork, and cheese. Sprinkle cilantro as desired. Add Cilantro Ranch Salad Dressing just before serving.

There is a restaurant chain called Café Rio Mexican Grill that has locations throughout Utah, Arizona, California, Colorado, Idaho, and Nevada. They serve a sweet pork salad that is tasty and popular. I've come up with a healthier version of this salad that tastes just as delicious.

Pork Ingredients:

pork sirloin tip roast, 2.5 lb.

1/2 cup salsa

1 1/2 cups peach or mango salsa (any fruited salsa)

1 cup chicken stock/broth

chipotle peppers in adobo sauce (add to taste)

2 limes

Lime Cilantro Rice ingredients:

1 tablespoon olive oil (optional)

2–3 cloves garlic, crushed (optional)

1 cup uncooked brown rice

2 cups chicken or vegetable broth or water

1/2 teaspoon salt

2 tablespoons fresh lime juice

zest from one lime (about 1/2 teaspoon or to taste)

1/4 to 1/2 cup cilantro, finely chopped

Salad ingredients:

5 to 6 cups Romaine lettuce, shredded or torn into bite-sized pieces

fresh cilantro, chopped

2 cups Lime Cilantro Rice

1 can black beans, rinsed well

2 cups roasted corn, warmed

1-3 avocados, slided

Shrerdded Pork

cheese, shredded or crumbled (Mexican blend or queso fresco)

Cilantro Ranch Dressing

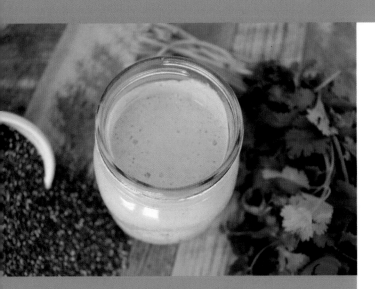

Directions

In a high-powered blender combine Greek yogurt, tomatillos, garlic, cilantro, hot peppers or red pepper flakes, lime juice, salt, and maple syrup or honey. Add chia seeds to thicken and blend in blender one more time. Refrigerate for at least 2 hours prior to serving.

Cilantro Ranch Salad Dressing

2 cups plain nonfat Greek yogurt

3 tomatillos

3 garlic gloves, crushed, or 1 teaspoon bottled garlic

1/2 bunch fresh cilantro, including stems (about 1/2 cup)

fresh hot peppers or red chili pepper flakes (to taste)

3 tablespoons fresh lime juice

1/2 teaspoon kosher salt

1 tablespoon real maple syrup or raw honey

2 tablespoons chia seeds

Nutritional Breakdown

For 1/8 of the pork salad (about 2 cups without salad dressing):

Protein 30.5 g, Fiber 5 g, Sodium 437 mg, Total fat 6.3 g, Saturated fat 1.9 g, Total carbs 30, Sugars 9.7, Calories 319 Kcal

For 1/3 of the Cilantro Ranch Salad Dressing (about 3 tablespoons):

Protein 14 g, Fiber 0.7 g, Sodium 98.7 mg, Total fat 0.5 g, Saturated fat 0.2 g, Total carbs 8.3 g, Sugars 4.6 g, Calories 63 Kcal

Chapter 8: Prepare Your Food

Visit FoodsWithJudes.com/book-content for recipes, articles and videos.

The Asparagus Revolution

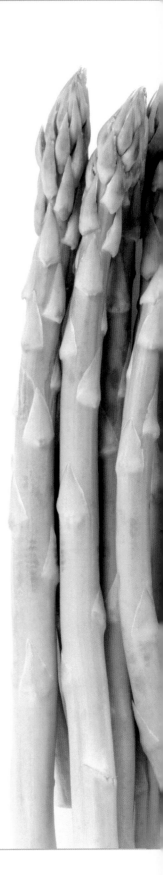

I was at my sister Janet's house once, chatting with her in the kitchen, when her husband, Randy, walked in the door holding a bundle of asparagus.

"Ugh," she said to him. "Why did you buy those?"

"I thought we could eat them with dinner tonight," he replied.

"No way," she said. Her nose wrinkled up. "I hate asparagus."

Surprised, I turned to look at her. "You can't be serious," I said. "How can you hate asparagus?"

"How can you like them?" she retorted. "They're so bitter and tough."

I took the bundle of asparagus out of Randy's hands. "Leave this to me," I said.

Right before dinner that night, I pulled a baking pan and some olive oil out of her cupboards. Then I spread all the asparagus spears out on the pan, drizzled the oil over them, tossed them until they were coated, and finally sprinkled them with sea salt. I put them in the oven at 425°F.

Ten minutes later, I was serving Janet roasted asparagus.
She took one bite and her eyes went wide. "These are amazing!" she exclaimed.

Shock was written all over her face. She'd been convinced that she hated asparagus for fifty years, only to discover that when they were prepared right, they were delicious.

Janet raved about those roasted asparagus all through dinner, and Randy was encouraged to bring them home more often.

Easy Prep Formulas

My sister's story is many other people's story, too. Healthy food might be great for you. It might deliver tons of nutrients, give you more energy, and make you feel and look better. If you don't know how to prepare whole foods fast and deliciously, none of that matters. It will take too much effort or won't taste good, and you won't end up eating it.

I myself spent years convinced that I hated Brussels sprouts. Then one night, I had a life-changing experience. Several years back, my foodie nephew, Matt, ordered Brussels sprouts at a restaurant for the table, and I tried one. They were absolutely delicious. I had just been preparing them wrong. Now, I cook a whole stalk of Brussels sprouts and eat them like candy.

Change can be difficult, especially when it comes to what you put in your mouth. My 12-FIX LEAN LIFE PLAN encourages particular types of foods that help us burn body fat, build muscle, decrease the damage of ongoing inflammation and stay healthy, full, energized, alert, and focused. I want you to be able to enjoy eating fruits and vegetables, yogurt, beans, lentils, whole grains, and fish.

I want to make your transition to these health-promoting foods as easy and scrumptious as possible. So easy, in fact, that you have nutritious ideas of what to fix even when you are rushed and frantically trying to get dinner on the table. You just have to be willing to make foods in new ways. I've included some simple formulas to make preparing these types of foods even easier. Start by choosing a few quick recipe ideas for your meals and snacks.

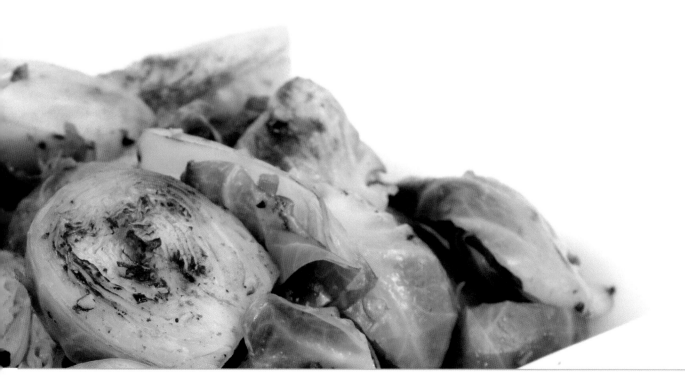

Fast and Delicious Vegetables

Many people complain about not liking vegetables. But when you cook them right, those complaints disappear.

You can transform your veggies into delicious delicacies in many different ways: shaving, spiraling, grilling, broiling, roasting, pureeing, stir-frying, blending, and tossing them. In this section, I'll take you through some of my favorite preparation techniques. Keep in mind that these prep methods work for many fruits as well!

Shave Your Vegetables

A smoother look and texture makes vegetables more appetizing. You can shave your vegetables lengthwise with a simple vegetable peeler to create flat, long-ribboned veggies that are enticing. Plenty of vegetables are great candidates for shaving. Try it with cucumbers, carrots, parsnips, zucchini, and other types of summer squash. You can toss shaved vegetables into a salad or sauté them into silky wide noodles.

Zucchini Ribbon Noodles

Spiral Your Vegetables

It takes just a few minutes to transform your vegetables into thin, uniformly curly spirals or long vegetable strands with a vegetable and fruit spiral slicer. When you do, you can create new looks and textures with almost any vegetable (or fruit) quickly with very little cleanup! Zucchini is the most popular vegetable to put through a spiralizer to make substitute pasta or noodles (zoodles), but don't stop there. Spiraled sweet potatoes make deliciously attractive noodles too. Add them to Asian soup for instance. Even spiraled rutabagas make great-tasting noodles. I love spiraled carrots and red peppers in my stir-fries and spiraled cucumbers, apples, and roasted beets in my salads. Roasted spiraled sweet potatoes or apples make the best kind of chips. Have fun with it!

Spiral Vegetable Salad

Grill Your Vegetables

A fantastic way to cook vegetables is to grill them. Grilling is one of my favorite ways to prepare veggies, because the slight charring brings out some delicious caramelized flavors in the food. Marinate the vegetables in high-heat oil mixed with herbs, garlic, or lemon juice for about an hour to help caramelize them, or coat them very lightly with olive oil using an oil mister. A combination of herbs and spices such as rosemary or thyme will make your vegetables stand out. Slice soft vegetables such as zucchini a quarter inch thick but harder vegetables thinner to prevent burning while cooking through. You really can't go wrong with this one!

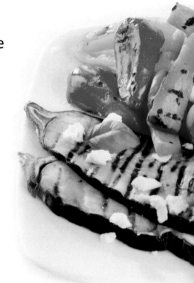

Grilled Eggplant

Broil Your Vegetables

If you're too busy to heat up the grill, just broil your soft vegetables for a similar caramelized experience in less time. Quickly cube vegetables and toss them in a bowl with vinaigrette or olive oil, salt, and pepper. Place them on a foil-covered pan about four inches from the heating element in your oven set on medium-high. Rotate, shake, or flip the vegetables to promote even browning while you stand guard to assess their cooking state. Make sure you keep an eye on them. Everyone has tried to leave for just a second and returned to burnt food!

Spicy Soba Noodles and Broiled Vegetables

Roast Your Vegetables

Roasting vegetables is incredibly simple. All you need is high-heat oil, salt, and a hot oven. The vegetables take almost no preparation, and they're delicious. Roasting brings out the natural sweetness in your vegetables. They become crisp and caramelized on the outside, but soft and juicy on the inside. Sweet potatoes, purple potatoes, carrots, red bell peppers, beets, onions, zucchini, butternut squash, mushrooms, cauliflower, broccoli, asparagus, Brussels sprouts: almost any vegetable you can think of, you can roast!

You can use a mister to spray the oil over your vegetables or toss them in a little olive oil (not extra-virgin), salt and pepper, and maybe balsamic vinegar in a bowl. Roast your vegetables in a hot oven, between 375°F to 450°F, until they're browned and tender.

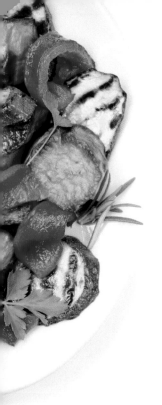

Dense, low-moisture vegetables such as root vegetables and winter squashes need the lower heat and more time in the oven, while vegetables with more moisture, such as eggplant or zucchini, need the higher end of this temperature range. The thicker the vegetable, the longer it will take to cook. Shake or turn the vegetables over halfway through to caramelize both sides. If they are tender but not charred, brown them with the broiler for a minute or two. Then pull them straight out of the oven and deliver them to the table. For an easy meal, top your roasted vegetables with a couple of fried eggs or a dollop of plain Greek yogurt seasoned with fresh herbs.

Devoured Vegetables

Puree or Cook Down Your Vegetables

Pureeing or cooking down your vegetables thickens and adds flavor to a dish. Root vegetables such as sweet potatoes and carrots, or winter squash, cauliflower, beans and lentils, or nearly any other vegetable can be added to your sauces, soups, and stews to cook down and thicken your recipes. You can add vegetable stock or water with onions and garlic to help the process get started if needed. You can speed up the process up by pureeing the vegetables (raw or cooked) and then adding them to your recipe. Skip thickening with flour, cornstarch, or arrowroot if possible and try adding vegetables to your recipe instead to add nutrition, flavor, and body at the same time! Try it with frozen or fresh fruit to replace syrup.

Yellow Lentil Vegetable Curry

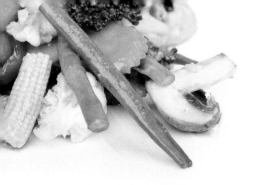

Stir-Fry Your Vegetables

Stir-frying is a tasty way to eat more vegetables, but I am often asked how to make the stir-fry sauce. The trick is knowing a few key basic sauce ingredients and then how to tweak the basic sauce recipe to make your favorite type of stir-fry. Combine your sauce with a variety of vegetables and protein choices you have on hand. Here's a simple formula for stir-fry sauce.

Basic Stir-Fry Sauce:

Shake or whisk to make basic stir-fry sauce. Choose a stir-fry flavor and make this stir-fry sauce come alive by following these flavor instructions:

- **Sesame Sauce:** Add 1 teaspoon sesame seed oil to the basic sauce.

- **Sweet & Sour Sauce:** Add 2 teaspoons tomato paste (double concentrated) + 3 to 4 teaspoons raw honey (or sugar) to the basic sauce.

- **Asian Lemon Sauce:** Reserve lemon zest of one lemon + replace rice vinegar with 1/4 cup lemon juice + 1 tablespoon raw honey (or sugar) + 1 teaspoon sesame seed oil added to the basic sauce.

Add stir-fry sauce of choice in this stir-fry formula.

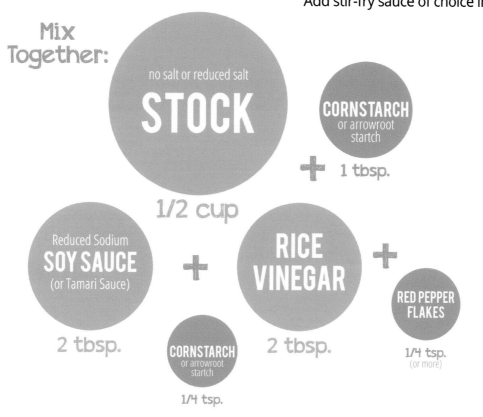

Basic Stir-Fry Sauce:

Mix Together:

no salt or reduced salt
STOCK
1/2 cup

CORNSTARCH or arrowroot startch
+ 1 tbsp.

Reduced Sodium **SOY SAUCE** (or Tamari Sauce)
2 tbsp.

+

CORNSTARCH or arrowroot startch
1/4 tsp.

RICE VINEGAR
2 tbsp.

+

RED PEPPER FLAKES
1/4 tsp. (or more)

Simple Stir-Fry Formula:

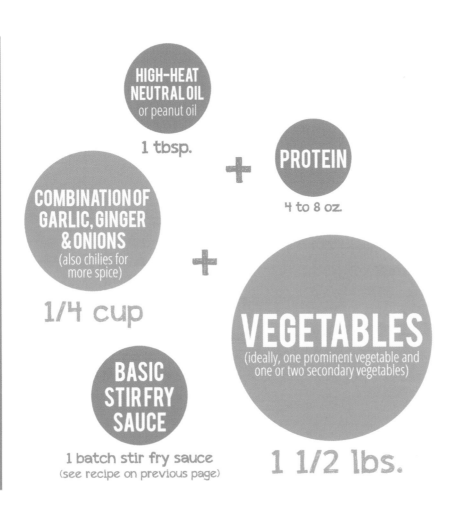

HIGH-HEAT NEUTRAL OIL or peanut oil

1 tbsp.

+

PROTEIN

4 to 8 oz.

COMBINATION OF GARLIC, GINGER & ONIONS (also chilies for more spice)

1/4 cup

+

VEGETABLES (ideally, one prominent vegetable and one or two secondary vegetables)

BASIC STIR FRY SAUCE

1 batch stir fry sauce (see recipe on previous page)

1 1/2 lbs.

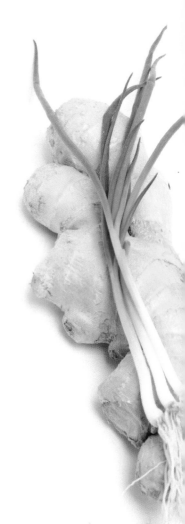

Note: If you use chicken in the stir-fry, marinate the chicken in egg white (1), sesame oil (about 1 teaspoon), cornstarch or arrowroot (about 1 tablespoon), and rice wine (enough to cover the chicken). Be sure to drain the marinade off before you cook it to help it brown.

Once your sauce is put together and the vegetables are cut, you are ready to go. Using a wok or large skillet over high heat, add any combination of garlic, ginger, and onions in hot high-heat safflower, canola, or peanut oil. Cook for about a minute while stirring. Add a protein (tofu, bean curd, chicken, shrimp, etc.) and stir-fry until browned (or pink for shrimp) and just cooked through. Remove protein to a plate and cover with foil. Add the thickest, densest vegetables to the pan first and stir-fry for a couple of minutes (you may need another teaspoon of oil if it is sticking). Then add thinner, faster-cooking vegetables. Stir-fry for about a minute. Add the sauce of choice and stir until tender but still crisp. Add the protein back in, heat through, and serve. Finish with a few toasted sesame seeds (optional) and serve with brown rice.

Simplified Stir-Fry Formula

Once you start preparing your vegetables in these tasty ways, you'll find that people eat a lot more of them.

Simple Salad Formula

A lot of people like green salads but don't prepare them often enough. That's unfortunate, because salads can deliver a big boost to your health! Making salads and salad dressings can actually be quick and simple. Follow this simple formula to add more salads to your life:

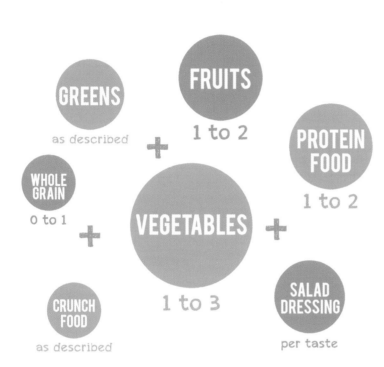

Simple Salad Formula:

GREENS *as described* + FRUITS 1 to 2 + WHOLE GRAIN 0 to 1 + VEGETABLES 1 to 3 + PROTEIN FOOD 1 to 2 + CRUNCH FOOD *as described* + SALAD DRESSING *per taste*

- **Greens:** I recommend crisp lettuce such as Romaine for at least some of the greens, and you can also add fresh basil, mint, or cilantro for extra flavor.

- **Vegetables**: Thinly sliced red onions are a great standard vegetable to add, along with others to suit your taste—even cooked ones! Roasted or grilled vegetables add so much to a salad. Marinated vegetables, like artichokes, work too.

- **Fruits**: Avocados are a great idea, and you can also add sweeter options such as pomegranates, pears, apples. oranges, or berries.

- **Protein:** Cheese, shelled edamame, chickpeas, lentils, and salmon are all great options, but any protein works. Try leftover protein from the previous night.

- **Whole Grains:** Larger, chewier grains such as farro and wheat berries are a great combination with salad. Red quinoa and black rice add color, but any whole grain works. While whole grains are optional, they do add another dimension to a salad that keeps you full longer.

- **Crunch:** For the "crunch food," toss in a few toasted nuts or seeds; avoid croutons! I usually buy my nuts already toasted from Trader Joe's, but it's to toast nuts up in a skillet. Sunflower seeds, hemp seeds, sesame seeds, pomegranate seeds are good ones to add.

- **Salad Dressing:** Finally, add a small amount of salad dressing to the dish just before you serve it. Go easy. You can add more if you need it. Strong cheese, some protein choices, and marinated vegetables add lots of flavor, so less dressing is needed.

Pomegranate Green Salad with Tuscan Pomegranate Vinaigrette

For More Basic and Delicious Salad Dressing Recipes

I have a quick and easy formula for salad dressing, too.

Add equal amounts of extra-virgin olive oil and balsamic vinegar. Infused extra-virgin olive oil and balsamic vinegars add even more flavor. Add an emulsifier such as mustard, tahini, plain yogurt, ground flax, ground chia seed, or mashed avocado to thicken. Add more emulsifier if you want the dressing thicker. Salt and pepper to taste. Shake to mix.

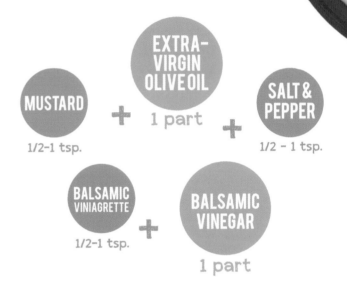

60-Second Salad Dressing Formula

MUSTARD
1/2–1 tsp.

EXTRA-VIRGIN OLIVE OIL
1 part

+

SALT & PEPPER
1/2 – 1 tsp.

BALSAMIC VINIAGRETTE
1/2–1 tsp.

+

BALSAMIC VINEGAR
1 part

 60-Second Salad Dressing

Optionally, you can top it off with 1 to 2 teaspoons of flavorings — dried herbs or seasonings, fresh herbs, crushed garlic, or shallots. Note: If you use another type of vinegar besides a balsamic dressing, the ratio to oil and vinegar changes to 1 part oil to 1/3 part vinegar.

 Guilt-Free Creamy Dressing

 Simple Asian Salad Dressing

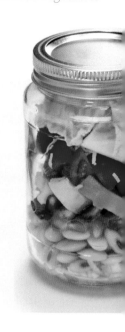

Mason Jar Salads to Go

Looking for an easy way to eat more salad on the go? Layer your salad into a wide-mouth mason jar or another similar container to keep the ingredients separate until you eat them. Premake your salads so that you're prepared to grab them and go when it's crunch time. Put your salad dressing and firmer vegetables at the bottom of the jar, giving the veggies time to marinate while your lighter, more fragile ingredients sit on top. Then just keep the jar upright until it's time to eat. Shake or stir it up, and enjoy!

Smoothie Bowl Formula

Smoothie bowls are a great way to boost your intake of fruits and vegetables. When a sweet treat is called for, they can definitely fit the bill. A good smoothie bowl is healthy, filling, and refreshing all at the same time.

This formula makes smoothies on the thicker side for the perfect smoothie bowl. Just pour your smoothie into a bowl and top with low-sugar granola, fruit, nuts, seeds, and fun surprises like unsweetened coconut. Chewing your food, rather than drinking it, may add to your level of satisfaction. Having nutritious, chewable food on your smoothie bowl allows your body to do more work breaking the food down. High fiber foods help slow down the digestion or the smoothie bowl and burn the calories more efficiently.

Smoothies made with yogurt can be a fantastic way to take in some extra protein and probiotics at breakfast. You can also sneak healthy foods into your smoothie that you don't normally like to eat. My favorite example is spinach. I slip spinach into fruit smoothies for my kids. Then I don't tell them that it's in there until they rave about how good the smoothie is. Even after they know that it's in there, it's so good that they don't seem to care. I have a formula for spectacular smoothie bowl. It goes like this:

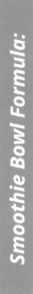
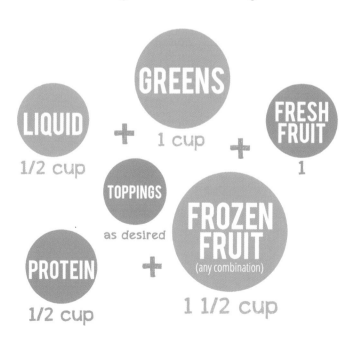

Smoothie Bowl Formula:

LIQUID 1/2 cup + **GREENS** 1 cup + **FRESH FRUIT** 1

TOPPINGS as desired

PROTEIN 1/2 cup + **FROZEN FRUIT** (any combination) 1 1/2 cup

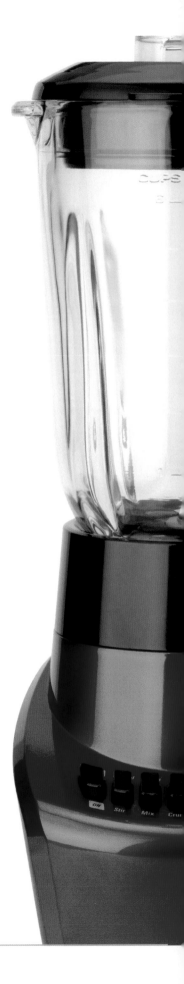

- **Liquid**: Your liquid can be milk, almond milk, pureed fruit, or 100 percent fruit juice.

- **Frozen Fruit**: Any unsweetened frozen fruit works, including puréed acai fruit. Using frozen fruit instead of ice gives the smoothie more flavor. Frozen fruit is always available and retains nutrients longer than fresh fruit.

- **Greens**: Smoothies are a great way to sneak veggies such as kale (with or without the stem), baby spinach, and Swiss chard into your diet.

- **Protein**: This can be yogurt, cottage cheese, silken tofu, nuts, peanuts, or nut butter. You can add a couple of tablespoons peanut butter powder or a protein powder, but I'm trying to encourage you to eat your food in whole food form so all the nutrients in that food can work together to improve your health.

- **Fresh Fruit**: Smoothies are also a great way to use up overripe fruit. If I see an apple or another fruit looking like its time has passed, in it goes. Fresh fruit adds some natural sweetness to the smoothie which is particularly important if the liquid you're using isn't fruit juice.

- **Toppings**: I'm talking about things like low-sugar granola, muesli, chocolate nibs, unsweetened coconut, pumpkin seeds, pomegranate seeds, berries and other diced fresh fruit, hemp seeds, chia seeds, ground flaxseeds, sunflower seeds, nuts or nut butters, and even yogurt.

Once you've gathered your ingredients, put them into a high-powered blender in the order listed in the formula to get the best smoothie results. If you want the smoothie thicker, add a tablespoon of chia seed and give it a couple of minutes. Add more fresh fruit or liquid if you like your smoothies thinner. Add a healthy sweetener (real maple syrup, pitted Medjool dates, etc.) to taste if you want it sweeter.

If you're going to make smoothies, it's best to invest in a high-powered blender. Regular blenders burn out fairly quickly when you use them a lot, and they function much more slowly when you throw in kale, spinach, and whole frozen fruits. Even though it costs more up front, you'll save more in the long run when you start blending your overripe fruits and veggies instead of throwing them out.

For Spectacular Smoothies: 6 Tips for Better Smoothies

Savory and Sweet Yogurt

Throw away the notion that yogurt is just for yogurt parfaits and smoothies. Savory or sweet, yogurt and kefir can be used in all sorts of ways to make food taste better and more nutritious! Both India and the Middle East have delicious, mild versions of cucumber yogurt that are wonderful on all sorts of foods, from spicy curries to chicken. Chicken marinated with yogurt remains juicy even if it is a little overcooked.

Greek yogurt replaces mayo and keeps food creamy and tasty when you add a vinaigrette to match the consistency you need. Try it in pasta, slaw, and chicken and tuna salads. I even add plain Greek yogurt to mashed potatoes to cream them up and add nutrition. Dips prepared with yogurt instead of mayo often taste better. Mix mashed avocados with yogurt for a delicious dip. Creamy salad dressings made with yogurt are outstanding and so much healthier. You can thicken or top with plain Greek yogurt instead of sour cream for soups, chili, salmon cakes, etc.

On the sweeter side, vanilla yogurt (or add pure maple syrup to plain yogurt), along with fruit, makes a wonderful topping for pancakes, waffles, and crepes. I love to bake with yogurt and kefir to add nutrition while cutting the butter. Plus, when kefir replaces buttermilk in baked goods such as muffins, quick breads, and pancakes, the consistency is silky and smooth. Add Greek yogurt to your ice cream maker. It's creamier and freezes faster than regular yogurt. The healthy bacteria will even survive a freezing.

Buy yogurt or make it. It takes only two ingredients, and you can do it right in a mason jar. Try it at least once to see how incredibly easy, economical, and especially delicious it is!

Let's Make Yogurt!

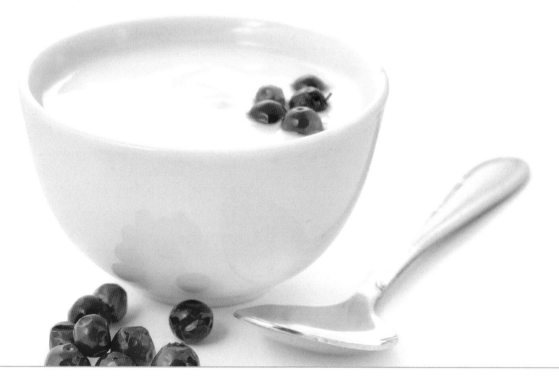

Don't Spill the Beans

I covered the bountiful benefits of beans and lentils in Chapter 2. Beans, lentils, and root vegetables thicken foods with flavor and nutrition. Beans can often be used to replace flour (1 cup beans for 1 cup flour) and meat in recipes. But how do you prepare them to make them easy and delicious?

Low-sodium canned beans work in a pinch. Make sure you rinse them at least twice before you use them. Or you can use this easy method to cook dried beans: put them in a slow cooker (one pound or less for a three-and-a-half-quart cooker or smaller; two pounds or more for a five-quart or larger cooker). Pour water over the beans until they are covered by at least two inches. For some extra flavor, you can add a slice or two of ginger or some fennel or cumin seeds to the mix. Cook on low overnight, and check in the morning to see if they need more cooking time. When they're done, discard the cooking water and store them. Your cooked beans will keep well in the fridge for a week or in the freezer for up to three months so you can have them on hand to add to whole grains such as brown rice or quinoa.

Dried lentils are perfect for rounding out green salads during hot weather and hearty soups and stews in the winter months. Regardless of the season, their quick-cooking, no-soak-required nature makes them ideal for hectic weeknight meals. Make extra lentils to add to other foods throughout the week.

Lentils cook much faster than beans and are a delicious way to thicken soups and stews while adding volumes of nutrition. Red, yellow, and orange lentils cook more quickly and add flavor and color to foods, but they tend to be mushy when heated—which makes them perfect thickeners. Green or

brown lentils, meanwhile, hold their shape better with heat.

Luscious Lentil Soup

The most reliable way to cook perfectly tender lentils is to bring them to a rapid simmer, and then reduce the heat to low for the rest of the cooking. They should cook with a few bubbles in the water and some gentle movement in the lentils. Try warm lentils tossed with good olive oil and vinegar with a cooked egg to complete the meal.

Another particularly delicious and nutritious bean is edamame. Edamame beans are simply unripened green soybeans. They have 30 to 45 percent more protein than other protein-rich members of the bean family, and unlike beans and lentils, this protein has all the essential amino acids.

You can purchase edamame frozen or already cooked, with or without the pods, and add them to your whole grains, salads, and stir-fries. They also make a wonderful high-protein snack: just cover and heat the edamame in the microwave. The beans slip right out of the pods and into your mouth; even kids have fun eating them. Best of all, there's no need to worry about negative health side effects, because it turns out that soy is exceptionally healthy, especially when it's unprocessed.

Read More About Soy

Beat the Rice and Pasta Rut

Are you in a rice and pasta rut, searching for ways to eat more whole grains? Start by adding beans, lentils, or edamame to rice and some of the whole grains listed in this section.

For a fun and nutritious whole grain, try wild, black, or red rice. Brown basmati rice smells like popcorn and has a nice flavor. Use a rice cooker to make it easier. Make the brown rice taste even better by using no-salt or low-salt stock instead of water. Or you can branch out beyond rice and pasta altogether. Whole-grain couscous and quinoa are particularly well-suited to substitute for rice, but most whole grains make delicious alternatives as well.

Black Rice Harvest

Don't be afraid to prepare whole grains. Most of them can simply be boiled like rice until they're tender. If they start to get too tender, drain the water off; if they're still not tender when there is no water left, just add a little more water. Bigger, chewier grains (called "berries") take about an hour to cook, but they hold their shape well.

Whole grains keep for about five days, so you can make them in advance and use them throughout the week by mixing them with beans, lentils, and other grains to shake it up. Try them in salads and soups and mixed together in different combinations. Try unfamiliar grains by mixing them in with a grain you are already used to eating.

My favorite whole grain is farro, which cooks in fifteen minutes flat and is both chewy and full of flavor. Kamut, sorghum (Wondergrain), spelt, black rice, wild rice, brown basmati rice, amaranth, and a type of young green wheat called freekeh are other delicious ways to free yourself from the rice and pasta rut.

Have you noticed how easy it is for some trendy, fast-casual restaurants such as Chipotle to throw together a burrito bowl in front of you? You tell them what you like, and they throw it in a bowl. The bowls are delicious and quick. You can make a variation at home for a super-easy meal. Use one to two whole grains as a base and then pile on a combination of toppings varying in textures and a balance of salty, sweet, and acidic flavors. Use my simple Grain Bowl Formula to get started.

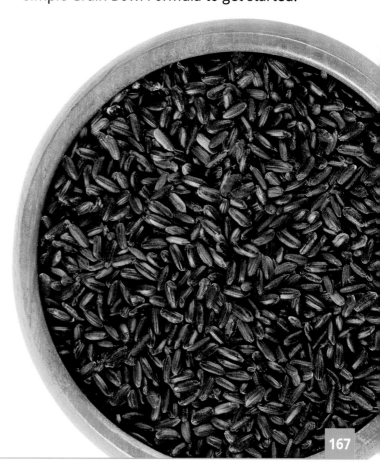

- **Whole grains:** Cooked whole grains such as sorghum; brown, black, red, or wild rice; quinoa; farro; barley; kasha; wheat berries; rye berries; Kamut; millet; amaranth; and freekeh go in the bowl first. Feel free to mix two or three different whole grains together.

- **Vegetables:** Any raw, steamed, roasted, marinated, sautéed, or pickled vegetable works. For heartier greens such as kale, collards, or cabbage, rub with a little vinegar to tenderize. Roasted vegetables, like Japanese eggplant, beets and broccoli, are magnificent in these bowls! As are lentils, chickpeas, beans, and dried peas of any sort, and pickled vegetables (such as kimchi or pickled cauliflower) or marinated vegetables such as artichoke hearts to adds lots of flavor to the bowl.

- **Protein:** Choose a creamy cheese such as ricotta or fresh mozzarella, poultry, pork, beef, lamb or fish (leftover or freshly cooked), eggs (over-easy, fried, soft boiled, poached, or scrambled), chickpeas, beans, lentils, dried peas, edamame, tofu, tempeh, or seitan. Smoked meats and strongly seasoned meats go a long way to add flavor to the whole bowl.

- **Fruit:** Avocado offers delicious creaminess, but other fruits add a bit of sweetness to balance the flavors. Pineapple, mango, pomegranate, papaya, chopped apples, pitted and sliced Medjool dates, and dried cranberries or cherries are a few ideas, but don't limit yourself.

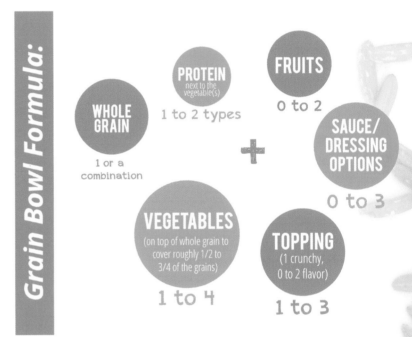

- **Sauce/dressing:** Olive oil, infused or regular balsamic vinegar, other types of vinegar, pesto, infused olive oil, vinaigrette, tahini sauce, sesame oil, peanut sauce, hoisin sauce, teriyaki sauce, fish sauce, tamari, soy sauce, tamarin, liquid amino, salsa, chutney, anchovy paste, chili-garlic sauce, gochujang (Korean chili sauce), harissa, Sriracha, miso, hummus, baba ghanoush, plain yogurt, fresh lime, or lemon can be used to add flavor and moisture to your bowl.

- **Toppings:** Preserved lemon; pickled vegetables such as pickled peppers or radishes; toasted seaweed; nutritional yeast; fresh herbs; cheese such as feta, goat, or Halloumi; chutney; and Kalamata olives add flavor, while sesame seeds, sunflower seeds, nuts, and pomegranate add crunch.

Build a Bowl: Easy Grain Bowl Formula

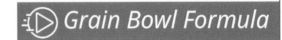 Grain Bowl Formula

Prepare to Eat Fish

Many people don't eat fish because they aren't sure how to prepare it. Don't let cooking fish scare you! It's so easy, and it can be much faster than chicken, pork, or beef. Here are five simple and delicious ways to prepare fish.

Broil Your Fish

This method is easy, fast, and tasty. Turn the broiler in your oven to high and cover a baking sheet with foil. Place your fish on the sheet, brush it with high-heat olive oil, add salt and pepper or a thin layer of miso paste or Dijon mustard, and slide the sheet pan into the oven so that it's about four inches below the heating element. The general rule of thumb is to cook the fish eight to ten minutes per inch of thickness (for quarter-inch fillets, it would be two to four minutes). When the fish is opaque and a knife slides easily into the thickest part of the fillet, it's done. Make sure you don't overcook it! Charred chopped tomatoes, ribboned summer squash, and red onion can cook with the fish on the same pan. Add capers to this vegetable mix and eat over the fish.

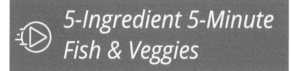 *5-Ingredient 5-Minute Fish & Veggies*

Easy Broiled Fish with Vegetables

Roast Your Fish

Roasting fish is similar to broiling it, but it takes a few minutes longer. Place the fish and a little oil on a hot, preheated pan or baking sheet and put it into a 450°F oven to cook. Salmon is good roasted in the oven with just a little olive oil, salt, and pepper, but you can also use any fresh herb mixture with reduced-salt tamari or soy sauce and real maple syrup, cooked down, reduced to a thicker sauce and brushed onto the salmon. Make your meal even easier by wrapping vegetables and fish together in foil.

Sesame Balsamic Salmon

Pan-Cook Your Fish

You can pan-cook fish in less than fifteen minutes. For thin fillets, try dredging the fish in sesame seeds or crushed nuts on both sides. Add to a large nonstick skillet over medium high heat with 1 to 2 teaspoons each of sesame seed oil and a neutral oil such as canola.

Cook for about two to three minutes or until seeds or nuts on the bottom are toasted and the top starts to turn opaque. Then cook on the other side one to two minutes. Add reduced-sodium soy sauce (with the sesame seeds) or salt and pepper. Keep in mind that the stovetop works best for fish that are on the thinner side, about a quarter inch thick or less, unless you take a tip from many restaurants that sear their fish in a pan on both sides and then throw it in the oven to finish the cooking.

Lemon Pasta with Caramelized Onions and Fish

Steam Your Fish

Try steaming your fish on top of vegetables. Start by sautéing garlic, onion, and some vegetables of your choice in a large skillet. Then add your fish—sprinkled with salt and pepper—onto the vegetables, five to ten minutes before they're finished cooking (depending on how thick your fish is). Add some liquid (such as a can of diced tomatoes and its juice), adjust the heat to a simmer, and cover the whole pan to steam the fish until it is opaque and a knife can easily cut into it. Finish the vegetables, stirring occasionally. Season with fresh herbs and salt and pepper to taste.

Steamed Fish on Vegetables

Grill Your Fish

Grilling fish is another mouthwatering option, particularly in the summer or on an indoor grill. Heat your grill until it is very hot, above 400 degree F, and mist or rub both sides of the fish with a high-heat oil and your favorite herbs and spices. Even using just oil with salt, pepper, and lemon tastes terrific. If there is skin on the fish, keep it on to help hold the fish together.

Sear each side. Continue cooking until the center's temperature reaches between 130 and 135 degrees F; it will continue to heat up to around 140°F while it rests. If you like your salmon on the rare side, take it off at 120 degrees F. Don't overcook it; the fish will dry out. For a fail-safe way to cook fish on the grill, wrap it in foil, alone or with vegetables. Don't forget to squeeze a little lemon onto the fish before serving and savor every bite.

Easy Grilled Fish

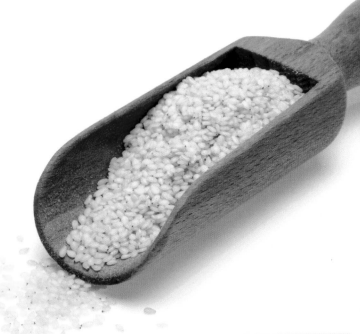

No-Mess Beet Avocado Salad

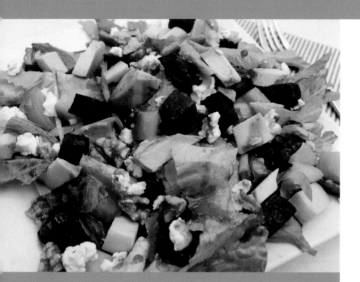

Directions

Preheat the oven to 400 degrees F.

Place washed and trimmed beets on a piece of foil. Wrap foil around each beet but before closing up the top and twisting, add a little high heat oil and a little salt and pepper. Roast until knife slices through beets easily, about an hour depending on the size of the beet. Beets can be cooked beforehand and kept in the refrigerator until you want to use them.

While beets are roasting, combine the balsamic vinegar, garlic, mustard and olive oil in a jar or bowl with a lid and shake. Season the vinaigrette, to taste, with salt and pepper.

While still hot and sitting in the foil, rub the skin with a paper towel and the skin will slide right off. Slice the beets into 1/4" pieces while still in the foil to alleviate any mess. Toss the cubes in a small bowl with enough vinaigrette to coat.

Combine greens, thinly sliced red onions, and avocado in a large bowl. Add crumbled goat or feta cheese and walnuts. Toss beets and dressing into salad just before serving. Enjoy!

This recipe is one of my all time favorite salads! I adore the delicious combination of roasted beets, avocados, greens, and goat cheese. However, beets can be so messy! My no-mess method to roast beets solves this problem. This gorgeous salad includes all of the amazing nutrition that beets, avocados, walnuts, and fresh greens offer for a super healthy lunch or dinner.

Ingredients

2 cups roasted and diced beets in 1/4" pieces (about two medium beets)

10 cups lettuce (mix a couple of varieties together), washed and torn

1/4 cup thinly sliced red onion

1 - 2 avocado, cubed and sprinkled with salt

3 ounces goats cheese (honey or regular), crumbled small

1 cup walnuts, toasted, coarsely chopped

Vinaigrette

1/4 cup balsamic vinegar

1/2 tsp crushed garlic

1/2 tsp mustard or tahini

1/2 cup extra-virgin olive oil

salt and freshly ground black pepper

Nutritional Breakdown

Protein 2.4 g, Fiber 2.6 g, Sodium 22 mg, Total fat 11.8 g, Saturated fat 0.8 g, Total carbs 6.3 g, Sugars 3.2 g, Calories 137 Kcal

Prosciutto-Wrapped Fish

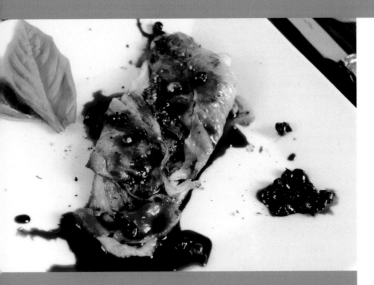

Chef Tim McCoy is the Educational Director of the International Culinary Arts & Sciences Institute, where I taught nutrition and healthy cooking. Chef Tim prepares this fast fish dish for his dad. With a few slight changes, he quickly makes a completely different fish recipe for himself (see below). When all is said and done, these two fantastic fish recipes are prepared in about fifteen minutes. Thanks for sharing, Chef Tim.

Ingredients

1 firm white fish fillet, 1/4 inch thick or less

1 or 2 fresh large basil leaves

1 slice of prosciutto

1/4 cup balsamic vinegar

1 tablespoon capers

Nutritional Breakdown

Protein 30 g, Fiber 0 g, Sodium 475 mg, Total fat 8.8 g, Saturated fat 0.8 g, Total carbs 10.4 g, Sugars 8.6 g, Calories 277 Kcal

Directions

Chef Tim takes a firm white fish fillet and places a fresh basil leaf or two to cover the top of the fish. Then he wraps the fish with one slice of prosciutto. Using a hot skillet sprayed with cooking spray, he sautés the wrapped fish over high heat on both sides for about two minutes or until the fish is opaque and a knife will slide into the fish without resistance. He finishes the dish by removing the fish from the pan. Then Chef Tim adds balsamic vinegar and capers to the pan. He reduces the vinegar over medium heat until it thickens to a syrupy sauce. He tops the fish with this sauce and some pepper. Yum!

Pan-Fried White Fish with Vegetables

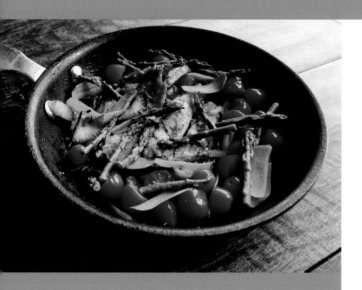

Tim McCoy is the Education Director of International Culinary Arts & Sciences Institute. He makes this quick fish recipe for himself. Thanks for sharing, Chef Tim.

Ingredients

1 firm white fish fillet, 1/4 inch thick or less

2 teaspoons high-heat oil, such as light olive oil or refined safflower oil

various vegetables such as sprouts, roasted asparagus tips, halved cherry tomatoes, julienned zucchini and carrot slaw, sautéed julienne peppers, arugula, or pea shoots

a couple of spritzes each of oil and vinegar

Nutritional Breakdown

One recipe:

Protein 28 g, Fiber 1.2 g, Sodium 378 mg, Total fat 21 g, Saturated fat 1.3 g, Total carbs 9 g, Sugars 4.7g , Calories 436 Kcal

Directions

For himself, Chef Tim skips the prosciutto and adds a little oil to the pan. He sautés the fillet on both sides over medium heat for about two minutes or until the fish is opaque and a knife will slide into the fish without resistance. After adding salt and pepper, he tops his cooked fish with various vegetables mixed with a little oil and vinegar. Fresh herbs, a pinch of your favorite spice, or just a squeeze of lemon or lime finishes the fish nicely too.

Chapter 9: Beyond Your Food

 Visit FoodsWithJudes.com/book-content for recipes, articles and videos.

Choose Your Own Adventure

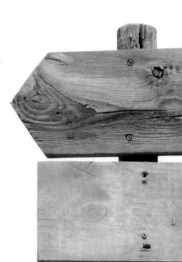

Your health is like a Choose Your Own Adventure book.

If you've never read one, the *Choose Your Own Adventure series* is a collection of books that all have multiple endings. You, the reader, arrive at your own ending or destination by the choices you make.

Let's say you're hiking through the Amazon jungle. You reach a point in the story where you come to a fork in the road, and you have two choices: Do you turn left, or do you turn right? Your decision leads you to a unique result at the end of the book.

Small is big. Over the months, years, and decades, those small choices turn into huge impacts on your weight and quality of life.

In one day you make about 250 food choices alone. Those are some of the forks in the road. Breakfast or no breakfast? What kind of snack do you eat as you rush out the door? Should you go ride your bike, or should you watch a TV show? Should you go to sleep now or keep surfing the net? You have the power to choose your journey by making small, seemingly insignificant healthy steps. You get to direct your own ending!

That's where exercise and sleep come into play. The amount and quality of each of these affect your food choices, muscle mass, strength, and overall health in a drastic way.

> In one day you make about
> 250 food choices alone.

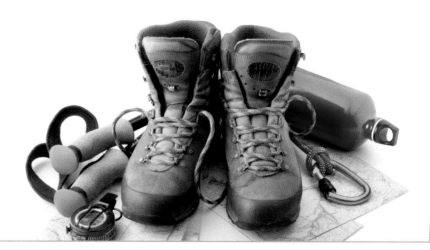

Movement and Sleep: As Important as Food

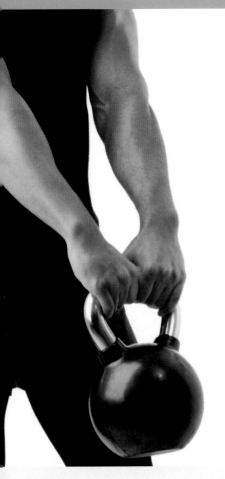

Movement and sleep are just as critical to your health as your food intake.

Have you ever noticed how difficult it is to resist nutrient-empty junk food when you're tired? Or how much easier it is to make positive food choices when you're rested? Movement and sleep, hand in hand, empower us to eat better, burn fat, and build muscle. When you get enough sleep and movement, you are energized and optimistic. You're happier, sharper, and more likely to make your health a priority and to find greater success in your work and relationships.

Keeping fat cells out of fat production mode has been a theme throughout this book and an important part of my fixes. As with food and beverage choices, exercise and sleep both have a positive effect on helping insulin in the body work more effectively. This means the insulin produced by the body works more efficiently, so less insulin is needed to do the same amount of work. That's great news, because many weight issues and type 2 diabetes are a result of insulin resistance. A rush of insulin tells fat cells to work overtime, sucking calories in and keeping those fat cells in lockdown mode. Using less insulin to do the same job makes a positive difference.

 # Think About It.

Movement and sleep are intertwined, enhancing each other. Consistent movement can be key to a better night's sleep. Regardless of age and demographics, movement has been consistently associated with better sleep more than any other behavior. The reverse is also true. We've all experienced the lack of energy and motivation that comes with a sleepless night. It's hard to be productive, much less to exert energy for a workout, without adequate sleep. With sleep, we can have more energy to move and enjoy doing it.

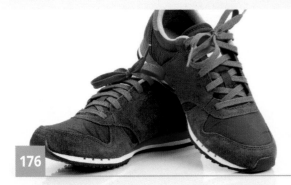

In this chapter, our fitness and wellness expert, Traci Fisher, will take you through the basics on how to make the most out of your movement regardless of your current activity level.

Move More by Traci Fisher

Move More. It really is that simple. This applies to everyone who is interested in living a healthy, strong life. "Move More" is a brilliantly simple way to summarize a potentially complicated subject. We have access to more resources than ever before. In an instant, we can access unlimited ideas on how to move, what not to do, and what we should do. It is literally endless, and can be absolutely overwhelming.

The word "Move" can mean many things: to pass to another place, proceed toward a certain state, to change position or posture. Our focus for movement is to not only do it, but to do it effectively. When you hear "Move," think quality. When you hear "More," think about building on that quality in a way that suits your lifestyle and goals.

We will explore the quality and quantity of movement and how both can be incorporated into your life anytime. When we aren't sure what to do amidst the mountain of information, we can simply return to the timeless guidance of this small phrase, "Move More." Let's get Moving!

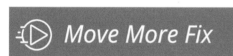 *Move More Fix*

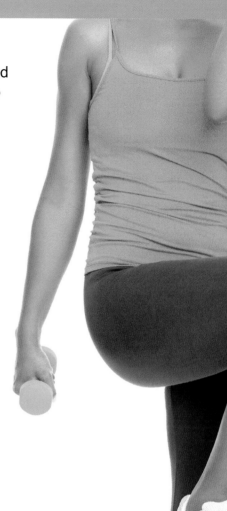

Our bodies are amazing machines! They move us through life, taking care of daily activities, keeping us upright in our chairs and cars, constantly taking in information, and processing it through our brains. Most of our daily movements are automatic – and we can thank the nervous system and its ability to adapt to our ever-changing environment without much thought on our part. We have major systems within our bodies that work together constantly, creating movement for us. In order to have optimal movement, we need to fuel our bodies with proper nutrition and rest. We also need to fuel them with effective and purposeful movement! Yes, the ways we move and the quality of that movement has a tremendous impact on our vitality. First, let's take a look at the power of movement and its impact on our lives.

The "Move" in Move More

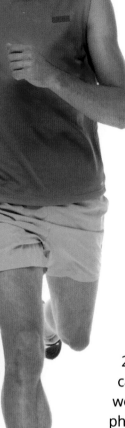

Why Move?

Our ability to move is one of the most important aspects of our existence. As we move, our bodies and minds benefit tremendously. A cascade of neurochemicals and growth hormones are released. Movement promotes brain cell repair, lengthens attention span, boosts decision-making skills and self-esteem, improves executive functioning, and prompts growth of new nerve cells and blood vessels. The mental and emotional benefits alone are worth the effort. Physical activity has been found to reduce cravings in alcoholics, treat depression, reduce symptoms in Alzheimer's patients, treat ADHD, and much more. We are wired to be rewarded chemically when we move.

Movement also has a multitude of physical benefits. It reduces the risk of many diseases and health conditions: cardiovascular disease, type 2 diabetes, metabolic syndrome, stroke, osteoporosis, and some cancers. We are discovering more evidence every day to prove what we already know: that moving feels good, mentally, emotionally, and physically.

 Did You Know?

We still have not uncovered all of the benefits of movement. Here are just a few:

- Helps manage chronic pain
- Wards off viruses
- Reduces risk of diabetes
- Reduces cancer risk
- Strengthens muscle
- Maintains mobility
- Improves coordination

- Strengthens bones
- Oxygenates the body
- Strengthens the heart
- Clears arteries
- Detoxifies the body
- Improves complexion
- Decreases risk of heart disease

A simple definition of movement is changing state, position, or place. With physical movement we can literally see a change in position or place. Movement also includes changes in states that we cannot always see, but that are just as vital to our health. Movement is dependent upon major systems within our bodies to include the muscular, skeletal, nervous, cardiovascular and respiratory systems. Optimal movement occurs when we are able to efficiently and effectively utilize our systems across the entire spectrum of movement. The "Move" in Move More encompasses this entire spectrum of movement and broadens our definition of what it means to move!

Human Movement System

The health of our movements are dependent upon major systems in our bodies. The Human Movement System (HMS) is made up of the muscular, nervous, and skeletal system. The HMS utilizes these 3 different systems in an intricately interwoven way to create movement. The nervous system acts on the muscular system to contract muscles; the muscular system acts on the skeletal system to create movement; and the skeletal system acts as a protective case for the nervous system. The system is known as the Kinetic Chain.

The support system for movement is the cardiovascular and respiratory system (cardiorespiratory system). As we move, our breathing and heart rates vary, depending on how much energy we need to complete the movement. How hard our heart has to work (heart rate) to achieve a certain movement is a strong indicator of the health of our bodies and hearts. All of these systems complement, support, and protect each other. We are able to twist and turn, run, jump, and enjoy deep breaths because of these systems. They are fueled with energy through nutrition, rest and, yes, movement!

Our bodies have to move for fuel as well. The most basic and subtle level of movement is in our bodies' supportive systems. Digestion, respiration, sweating, dilation, and constriction of blood vessels are just a few of the types of movements that occur beneath the surface. When we move physically, we are supporting all of our systems. Movement is a source of fuel in and of itself. So, of course, we want to ensure we keep moving for as long as possible. One of the ways to do that is to start with a strong foundation of proper movement mechanics and then build upon that.

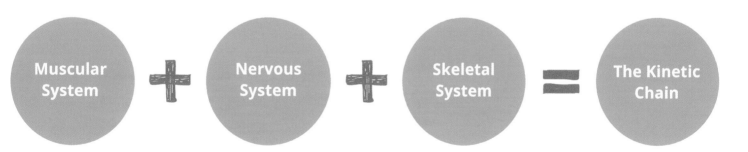

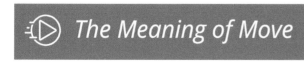

The Meaning of Move

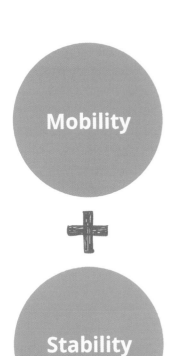

Movement Spectrum

The Movement Spectrum is based on both mobility and stability. Mobility is the ability to produce a desired movement, and stability is the capacity to resist an undesired movement. When we are able to stabilize our joints, ligaments, and muscles in an organized way to produce full mobility, then we have optimal movement.

Think of how your body moves on a roller coaster ride. If we didn't provide some internal resistance, we would be tossed around too much, so we "brace" ourselves to resist movement. As we brace, we are creating stability. It's not visible, but even as we are stepping out of the ride, we are still stabilizing some parts of our body while mobilizing others just to keep our balance. Our bodies are constantly stabilizing and mobilizing to maintain equilibrium.

This is exciting news if you don't feel ready to start an exercise routine. You can focus first on the quality of movement without having to worry about increasing quantity. Because sometimes getting moving can conjure up images of endless hours running or working out in the gym, motivation can fizzle. It is refreshing to know that just by focusing on the quality of movement, we are making a tremendous impact on our health.

 The Movement Spectrum

 Stability and Mobility

Your Movement

So, the focus of "Move" is quality. Quality movement occurs when our bodies' systems work together efficiently and effectively, in all types of environments, and across the entire spectrum of movement. So, how do we know if that is happening?

An easy way to determine the quality of movement is to take a look at our own stability and mobility. Stability and mobility include balance, coordination, flexibility, strength, and muscular endurance. There are many ways to test your quality of movement. The easiest is to take a look at current movement patterns, as well as aches and pains. If you are in pain, your body is talking to you. Make sure that you listen! We want to use all information, including pain, to assess the quality of our movements. If we have full range of motion at our joints, good posture, a strong center of gravity, stability during movement, and enough strength and endurance to complete the tasks that are important to us, then we are on our way to quality movement!

There are many ways to improve the quality of your movement. Focus first on improving the movements that are closest to the center of your body. Think of your lower back (stability), pelvis (mobility), upper back, shoulder, and chest (thoracic mobility). Your shoulder blades need to be stable to support all of the movement at your shoulder. Once your body is stable in the right spots, you can teach your body to move and balance as a whole. The fastest way to improve is to practice whole movements (check out our *"Improve Your Move"* video) with proper form. If there is a movement that you cannot perform, practice that exact movement in a controlled environment with support like a chair. Then, slowly, as your body learns, take away that support. Remember, quality first, then quantity!

 Check Your "Move"

 Improve Your "Move"

 Balance

 Flexibility and Range of Motion

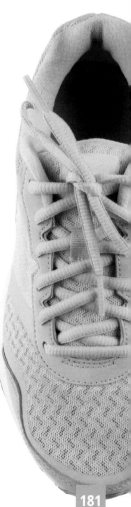

The "More" in Move More

If we want to counteract the process of aging and keep enjoying the benefits of movement, then we have to strive for More. Why? Because we have amazing bodies that thrive on being challenged. This is called specific adaption to imposed demand, which means that the human body is designed to adapt to any stress placed upon it. Over time, our bodies learn and certain movements no longer take as much energy—mentally or physically. This is a cool feature that comes with our bodies and allows us to adapt to and overcome our environment.

Why More?

Our bodies' ability to learn and adapt has served us well across the years. We used them to hunt, farm, build homes and move in many ways to protect ourselves and to stay alive. We evolved and we are still evolving - just in different ways. Now, we still need to Move to survive. And, since our bodies are built to adapt, that is exactly what they do.

As we spend more time hunched over our desks and less time upright and moving, our bodies adapt accordingly.

Some muscles work overtime while others are underworked. This can cause aches or injury and eventually leads to muscle imbalances and a host of other physical issues.

The positive news is that your body's ability to adapt to stress never goes away. As you change and challenge yourself, your body becomes more efficient and stronger and the benefits of moving add up. Better yet, this includes any change at all—even changes that seem insignificant. That's why we want you to Move, and to Move More!

 The Meaning of More

More can be defined in terms of the **type** of movement, **intensity** of movement and the amount of time spent moving both in terms of **frequency** (how much per week) as well as how much **time** spent on the activity each day. An easy way to remember how to add More is by thinking FITT: Frequency, Intensity, Time and Type. Moving our bodies should also be fun. Moving makes us feel alive.

Whether you are working on the quality of your movement, increasing the quantity, or both, your body begins to change whether you see it or not. Keep in mind that just by improving the quality of your movements, through adding balance, stability and mobility, you are already adding More.

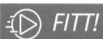 FITT!

F Frequency	The American College of Sports Medicine (ACSM), Centers for Disease Control and Prevention, and American Heart Association all have recommendations regarding the frequency, intensity, time, and type of movement that supports optimal health. The recommendations vary based on age and current levels of fitness but in general they recommend at least 150 minutes of moderate intensity activity OR 60-75 minutes of vigorous activity per week. They also recommend at least two days of strength and endurance activities. Keep in mind that these guidelines are goals for basic health. We want you to start where you are and then progress from there.
I Intensity	
T Time	
T Type	

Type of Movement

Twist, turn, dance, sprint, bend, reach, jump, spin, sit, contract, lift, exhale, stabilize; These are all great movements. Whatever type of movement you choose to engage in, first and foremost, it should have quality. We said that we can define quality of movement through the variables of mobility and stability. We asked, "How are you moving?" Many people may suspect that they need more balance, coordination, endurance, strength, or flexibility. Take a look at your physical history. If you have common injuries or aches, focus on stability and mobility first.

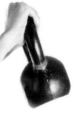

Time and Frequency of Movement

You can increase the quantity of your movement through time and frequency. Time refers to the amount of time spent doing an activity and frequency refers to how often an activity is done. For example, you can set a timer while working at your desk to remind yourself to stand up every hour (frequency) for a minute (time). Or if it suits you better, stand up every 90 minutes (frequency) for several minutes (time). The old boring suggestions, to park a little further away or to take the stairs, actually do make a difference!

Improving the quality of your movement (range of motion, balance, and some muscular imbalances) actually takes no extra time at all. For example, if you have already figured out that you need a bit more balance in your life, try standing on one foot while you engage in everyday activities like brushing your teeth, standing in line, or doing the dishes. You can also use this time to check out your range of motion just by literally moving your body at its joints - arm circles, neck rotations, hip circles, the options really are endless!

 More Type of Movement

Perhaps you are spending too much time hunched over at your desk and your shoulders are starting to bend a little too far forward. Every time you get up from your desk, reach back behind you, clasp your hands together and lift your chin towards the sky.

 More Time (and Frequency)!

Don't Have Time?

Here are some quick fixes you can use to "Move" a little "More" than you did yesterday:

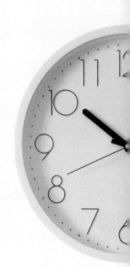

- Squeeze your butt muscles 3-5 times at every red light.
- Don't sit on the toilet; squat over it.
- Hold groceries, your cell phone, purse and dog leash with the opposite arm.
- Stand on one foot while brushing your teeth.
- Do a counter push up every time before you open the refrigerator.
- Park farther away than you did yesterday.
- Take the stairs at work, at the hotel, at the mall . . . everywhere!
- Every time you answer the phone, stand up and walk around.
- Set a timer to stand up and move around at least five minutes per day.
- Breathe very deeply as often as possible!

Intensity of Movement

Don't let this word scare you. Intensity is progressive and starts wherever you are. Increasing the intensity of an activity can mean doing more of it (frequency, time, type) or increasing the exertion or effort that you are expending. We have all seen the gadgets available to help us measure our intensity. But don't forget that your brain and heart are useful tools too. As you begin to exert more effort, your body knows it.

You know if a box is getting heavy or if the light bulb you are replacing above you is starting to feel like it has quadrupled its weight. This is called your rate of perceived exertion. Sometimes this happens naturally, and sometimes we make it happen on purpose.

For cardiovascular endurance, you can obviously increase the intensity by doing a movement more often or faster. We can also increase the intensity by moving different planes of motion. If you like to speed walk, turn sideways for part of the walk. Fortunately, it's really easy to increase intensity and we can do it pretty quickly.

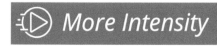 *More Intensity*

You define what "More" means to you. We all have different circumstances, capabilities, time, and, bodies. For some, moving more is standing up several times throughout the day at their desk. For others, it's completing a physical therapy exercise or getting into a strength training program. It could mean something completely different to you. The bottom line is to take a look at how you are currently moving and see how you might add "More" in a way that supports what you need.

This brings us to the Move More Formula. Personalize it by thinking about YOUR ideal weekly movements. Now think about your current movements in terms of its quality and quantity. This table combines Move and More across the entire spectrum of movement. Use it to increase your awareness of your current movements and how you might add a little More to get to your ideal movement pattern.

Type of Activity	Days per week (frequency)	TIme (spent doing the activity)	How hard you are working (intensity)	Fun! (do you enjoy this movement?)
Stability: Balance/Posture				
Mobility: Range of Motion/Flexibility				
Strength				
Cardiovascular				

 Your Move More Formula

FIX #11

Move More

This fix is called Move More. The "Move" in Move More ultimately means quality movement. Quality movement is the foundation for all other movement and is based on stability and mobility. That means that your body can stabilize itself in some ways while at the same time mobilizing in other ways. Think of the balance required on a step ladder as you rotate your shoulder to twist in a light bulb. You need both mobility and stability to do this safely.

Another way to see the quality of your movement is to pay attention to your posture, balance, and ability to have a full range of motion at all of your joints. If you know that you are limited or have recurring aches and pains, you need to address them first. It doesn't take any extra time to incorporate proper movement into the movements you already make every day. Try moving in the opposite way that you normally do. This can mean looking up towards the sky before looking down at your phone or contracting your back muscles at your desk. Become aware of how you move every day and make sure that you focus on adding quality to your current movements before you add quantity.

Quantity is where the "More" of Move More comes in. A way to do this is by applying the FITT (Frequency, Intensity, Time, Type) principle to your movement routine. Changing up any one of these variables means adding "More" to your "Move". Think about how you are currently moving. If there are any challenges to your balance, posture or stability, incorporate an activity that will strengthen those areas first. Just by focusing on the quality of movements, you'll already be doing "More" by increasing the variables of type, and frequency. Adding intensity and time can mean speeding up, moving in different directions, adding more weight, working out for longer—the options are endless.

"Move More" is simple, but that does not mean it is easy. As with all of the fixes in this book, our internal and external environments affect our choices. Here are some quick tips on how to make "Moving More" a reality that you can build on—starting right where you are.

1. Make it fun and make it yours! Moving our bodies should feel good. Discover how you like to "Move", whether it is gardening, golfing, walking around the mall with a friend, sightseeing, or discovering new group fitness classes in your area. Choose someone you want to strengthen your relationship with and ask them to join you.

2. Use the LEAN BODY, SMART LIFE app to share your progress. Fit movement into your life instead of trying to fit your life into a program.

3. Partner up! Accountability may sound intimidating, but it works. Find someone, like family members, friends, or coworkers. If you prefer to workout alone but still want some accountability, find someone you don't know in an online program.

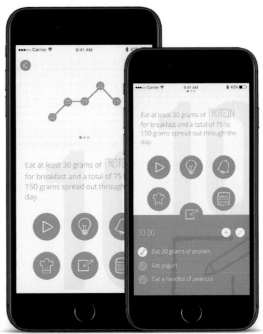

4. Start small! Yes, all of those little tips about parking farther away from the building, taking the stairs, and holding groceries instead of using a cart add up. Be creative and clever in your own life and see how you can move more by choosing different habits. (Stop parking the car at your mailbox to get the mail!)

5. Track it! The number one tip for increasing fitness levels is to track. Track using pen and paper or the LEAN BODY, SMART LIFE app. The simple act of tracking automatically creates awareness and results.

You now have a simple way to think about and break down what it means to Move More. Regardless of your current activity level, age, or circumstances, remember that your body is the most amazing machine on this earth. Take a fresh look at how you Move and do not let anyone else tell you what you "should" be doing. Define your own ideal movement patterns and go for it.

Remember, exercise is optional, but movement is mandatory. Keep challenging your body. Create the adventure you inherently deserve!

Fix #11 Action Plan:

✓ *Choose new ways of moving to incorporate into your daily life. Take the stairs instead of the elevator, stand on one foot, stretch every time you stand up.*

✓ *Think of a type of movement that you really enjoy like dancing, tennis, or gardening, and make time for it!*

✓ *Use the Movement Formula Table to see where you can add in a little More frequency, intensity, time or type of movement!*

✓ *Whatever exercise you do, write down the specifics at least one time. One month later, do it again and see how much you have improved.*

✓ *Check your current workout plan to see if you are hitting all the elements of a well-rounded program: strength, cardiovascular, coordination, balance, and flexibility. If you're not, replace one session with another type of training.*

✓ *If you are rushed or less motivated on any given day, have a shorter, easier exercise plan as a backup plan rather than forgoing all your exercise that day. It might be as easy as walking or jogging a short distance.*

✓ *Regardless of your current activity level, check the quality of your movement to ensure that your body is in alignment, regardless of your current activity level.*

Track Your Progress on The LEAN BODY, SMART LIFE App

Snooze to Lose

Sleep can be medicine or poison.

The first eleven fixes introduced as part of the 12-FIX LEAN LIFE PLAN are all about making small changes for a big return. Sleep is no different. Somehow, it has become a badge of honor in our society to get by on less sleep. Yet the bottom line of your health and success is directly related to the amount of sleep you get. Getting enough sleep ensures that you have sufficient energy to live to the fullest. When you have energy from a good night's sleep, you tend to make wiser choices with your movement and

nutrition. The length and quality of your sleep has a direct impact on how you experience life. When you have enough sleep, you improve your memory, spur creativity, sharpen your attention, and improve your motivation and performance. You also improve your long-term health with enough sleep. Chronic inflammation, insulin resistance, and obesity all improve with sleep. Sleep directly affects your muscle and body fat levels. If you snooze, you lose!

Memory, Creativity, Concentration, Motivation, Performance

Sleep plays an important role in memory, both before and after learning. Both the quantity and quality of sleep affect learning and memory. Without sleep, you cannot focus your attention enough to learn or unify new information well enough to remember it. It's harder to learn and retain information. With sufficient sleep, you can consolidate memories and make them stronger. The emotional components of memory are also strengthened during sleep, which may help the creative process.

Lack of sleep can result in inebriated-type symptoms. Sleep-deprived individuals find it more difficult to concentrate, assess situations, and make decisions. Lack of adequate sleep even affects mood, motivation, judgment, and our perception of events. Without enough sleep, life seems harder. Lack of sleep contributes to depression, irritability, moodiness, and anxiety.

Muscle and Body Fat

Skipping out on adequate sleep can lower your muscle mass and can result in extra visceral fat around your middle. During sleep—particularly REM sleep—your body repairs and builds muscle while also breaking down fat for energy. Without enough quality sleep, you aren't able to build as much of that valuable muscle or burn as much fat. If you are up and not sleeping, you are more likely to eat late into the night, compounding the problem, leading to more nutritionless calories and less opportunity for your body fat stores to be used.

Several studies have investigated why we tend to eat more when tired. Lack of sleep often causes hormone imbalances that affect us negatively. These studies have found a strong relationship between the activity of the hunger hormone (ghrelin) and the number of hours of sleep. Furthermore, without enough sleep, the fullness hormone (leptin) levels drop while hunger hormone levels increase.

Given the hormone imbalance, it's not surprising that we eat more when skimping on sleep and significantly increase the number of calories we consume. A small study out of the Mayo Clinic found that sleep-deprived individuals may eat more than five hundred extra calories per day compared with people who get enough sleep. Researchers concluded that the sleep-deprived individuals ate more because tired people are often dysphoric, or unhappy, which makes them prone to food cravings—especially for foods high in carbohydrates and sugars.

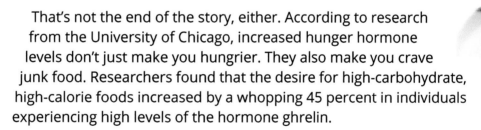

Your stress hormones are also affected by your sleep habits. Deep sleep neutralizes stress hormones, but lack of sleep triggers the release of stress hormones such as adrenaline and cortisol, increasing the risk of heart disease, belly fat, and muscle breakdown. Because stress hormones increase fluid retention, you can actually gain two pounds in body fluids from just one night of poor sleep.

That's not the end of the story, either. According to research from the University of Chicago, increased hunger hormone levels don't just make you hungrier. They also make you crave junk food. Researchers found that the desire for high-carbohydrate, high-calorie foods increased by a whopping 45 percent in individuals experiencing high levels of the hormone ghrelin.

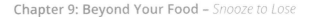

Other sleep studies using brain imaging found that the reward-seeking portion of the brain is stimulated by fewer than seven hours of sleep per night, increasing your desire for refined-carbohydrate foods that spike blood sugars and call for insulin. Insulin in turn drives calories into fat cells and keeps them there. Then your body craves more refined, processed foods, and the cycle of building body fat continues. Obesity, inflammation, and insulin resistance contribute to poor health.

Not only does lack of sleep compromise your immune system, making sickness harder to fight, but you may not recover as quickly, either. Too little sleep reduces cytokine production, which reduces the immune response to infection.

Sleep is central to your ability to keep fat weight off, function well, and be productive. For most of us, it's a matter of making it a priority. All you need to do is sleep seven or eight hours. If you can plan ahead to go to bed at an earlier time most nights, you can reap all of the many life-enhancing benefits that a full night of sleep has to offer.

The simple yet powerful act of sleep can enhance or sabotage your health and your success. In fact, all aspects of our lives are affected, so let's choose wisely.

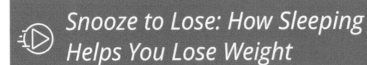

Snooze to Lose: How Sleeping Helps You Lose Weight

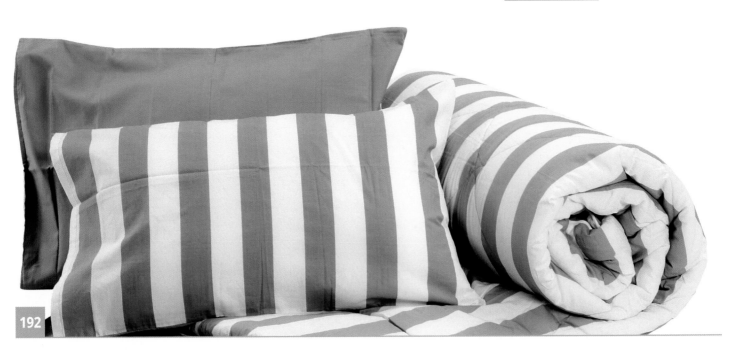

FIX #12

Sleep Seven to Eight Hours Every Night

Make sure to get between seven and eight hours of sleep every night. Set a time to go to bed, and stick to it. The hardest part of this fix is developing the discipline to turn off the TV or the computer screen at the end of the night. Blue-light screens from smartphones and computers right before bed are especially problematic for sleep. This kind of light sends the same signal to your body as sunlight, so your entire sleep cycle ends up delayed into the next morning. There is a function on some smartphones that can dim the phone automatically and use non-blue light on a schedule.

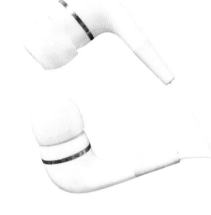

Leaving the phone in another room and getting a good old-fashioned alarm clock isn't a bad idea either. Kids and teenagers especially should be leaving their phones in rooms other than where they sleep at night.

Avoid eating at night, especially foods that are high in carbohydrates and sugars. These foods raise your blood sugar level and keep you from sleeping well. Additionally, stop eating early in the evening so that you are burning fat longer during the night. As discussed in Chapter 6, eating plenty of protein during the day boosts your levels of sleep-friendly hormones such as melatonin and serotonin.

As much as you may want to drink caffeine during the day to wake up, research indicates that it's part of the sleep problem in our country. Those who consume caffeine during the day sleep less with less sleep quality and have more daytime sleepiness than do their non-caffeine-consuming counterparts. That holds true for children, teenagers, and adults, so don't be misled by the influx of caffeine-packed drinks available now.

If you're not tired near bedtime, engage in some relaxing activities that put you in the mood to sleep. Read a book, listen to relaxing music, or meditate. Keep lights low or off if possible. Try smelling lavender essential oil; it can help you relax in preparation for sleep. Sleep in darkness, and keep the temperature in your room lower than 70°F when possible. If you have pets, try to keep them off the bed or out of the room so that they don't disturb you.

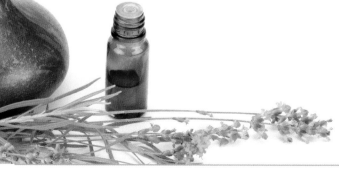

Fix #12 Action Plan:

✓ *Sleep seven to nine hours during the night as often as possible. Make it a priority!*

✓ *Stay away from blue-light screens at least two to three hours before going to bed, or change the screen to white light.*

✓ *Turn off phones, computers, and TVs during the night.*

✓ *Keep lights dim or off during the hour prior to bedtime, and block noise using earplugs.*

✓ *Turn down the thermostat when possible, as a cool room promotes deeper sleep.*

✓ *Get completely ready for bed at least one hour before bedtime and read, write, etc.*

✓ *Stick to a relaxing ritual prior to sleep.*

✓ *Resist the temptation to squeeze one more task into the end of your day.*

✓ *Avoid eating during the evening hours after a light dinner. If you do need to eat something, avoid sugar and refined carbohydrates.*

✓ *Over time, decrease your caffeine intake during the day.*

✓ *Infuse lavender essential oil in your bedroom or place some on a tissue and tuck the tissue into your pillowcase prior to bedtime.*

✓ *Keep pets off the bed during the night.*

Track Your Progress on The LEAN BODY, SMART LIFE App

Chocolate Protein Peanut Butter Shake

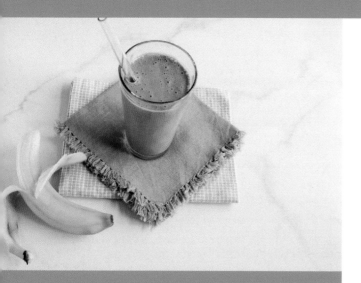

Directions

Place all ingredients in a blender, puree until blended, and serve immediately before it melts. Makes 2 cups. Enjoy!

This thick, cold chocolate peanut butter shake, made without the artificial taste of protein powder, is delicious and perfect for a snack, dessert, or post-workout. It's hard to believe that it's not a decadent ice cream shake. It contains thirty-five grams of high-quality protein using whole foods rather than protein powders. The bananas must be firmly frozen so the shake will be cold and thick. In fact, I pull the bananas out of the freezer right before putting them in the blender, so they don't have a chance to thaw. Whenever my bananas are beginning to get overripe, I quickly peel and slice the proper amount for my recipe and put them in the freezer for a future batch of this yummy shake. Shelled hemp seed is optional and doesn't affect the taste or the consistency, but it does add ten grams of plant-based protein, as well as omega-3 and omega-6 fats and other great nutrients. Enjoy!

Ingredients

1/2 to 2 tablespoons real maple syrup

1 tablespoon cocoa

4 tablespoons natural peanut butter

1 large or 2 small bananas, peeled, sliced, and frozen until firm

1 cup milk

3 tablespoons shelled hemp seeds (optional)

Nutritional Breakdown

For whole recipe without hemp:

Protein 26 g, Fiber 12 g, Sodium 207 mg, Total fat 34 g, Saturated fat 5.7 g, Total carbs 68 g, Sugars 61 g, Calories 657 Kcal

ckwheat Granola

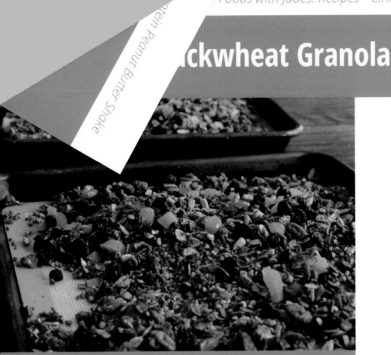

It's hard to buy granola this good and this healthy. My guru granola friend who pays ten bucks for a little bag of his special granola says that this granola is much better. It's full of protein and whole grains, including buckwheat. Even better, it's gluten-free as long as you use gluten-free oatmeal, and it's perfect eaten with yogurt or oatmeal.

Ingredients

2 cups old-fashioned oats

2 cups shredded unsweetened coconut

4 cups nuts and seeds like sliced almonds, pecans, roughly chopped, sunflower seeds, chia seeds, hemp seeds, etc.

1 cup raw or roasted buckwheat (kashi)

1/4 cup refined safflower oil, canola oil, or unrefined, cold-pressed coconut oil

1/2 cup raw honey (not for babies under one year old)

1/4 cup maple syrup

3 tablespoons cinnamon

1/4 to 1/2 teaspoon salt (optional)

3 cups dried fruit like cherries, cranberries, blueberries, apricots (chopped), etc.

Nutritional Breakdown

For 1/28 of this recipe (about 1/2 cup):

Protein 6.3 g, Fiber 5.0 g, Sodium 24.1 mg, Total fat 16.1 g, Saturated fat 5.7 g, Total carbs 27.4 g, Sugars 12.3 g, Calories 270 Kcal

Directions

Preheat oven to 325°F. In a large bowl, add the oats, coconut, a variety of nuts and seeds, and buckwheat. Mix together. In a small saucepan, heat and stir the oil, raw honey, maple syrup, salt, and cinnamon together. Pour one quarter of the heated mixture over the oat mixture and mix well. Continuing combining in small batches until both are mixed thoroughly.

Spread the mixture out onto a large jelly roll pan or baking sheet with a rim that is prepared with parchment paper or a nonstick silicone baking liner. Place in the upper portion of the oven, and every ten minutes use a large spatula to flip the granola to brown all sides. Cook for about thirty minutes or until browned through. When making a double batch, rotate the two pans every ten minutes when you mix or flip the granola because the top one browns. I cook them for forty minutes total when making two.

While the granola is baking, I mix the dried fruit together. After thirty to forty minutes, take the granola out of the oven and mix with the dried fruit. Let cool and store in airtight containers.

Chapter 10: Recipes For Success

12-FIX LEAN LIFE PLAN in Action

Recently, I married a wonderful man who definitely wasn't a "foodie," someone yearning for fresh, high-quality, and delicious food.

When we met, he was a business executive who didn't take much time for food and exercise. He ate out a lot, at both fast-food and sit-down restaurants filled with hamburgers, french fries, and steaks. At home, he ate his favorite go-tos: cereal every morning and plastic-wrapped American cheese slices toasted on white bread for lunch. He often ended his day with his biggest meal, quickly cleaning his plate even if he was full.

Over the first eight months and a lot of traveling, working, eating at restaurants, and activities, he moved more and made small, simple changes to what, how, and when he ate. He didn't diet; he slowly adopted the twelve fixes discussed in this book, little by little. He didn't apply the fixes all at the same time, but he began forming better habits without really trying. There was no dieting all-or-nothing mentality, so no deprivation either.

My husband was surprised that after many years of testing positively for high cholesterol (LDL), his LDL blood levels dropped within the normal range. After just nine months of following some of the twelve fixes some of the time, he had made a real difference to his health.

While his weight on the scale remained about the same, his waist size steadily diminished. My husband was amazed as he continued to move his belt notches down until, finally, he was forced to get a new belt. He went down a full pants size in eight months, having made many little changes but without the usual pain of dieting.

The food we ate was tasty and healthy, and we didn't spend much time in the kitchen making it. Don't think I was always cooking for him, either. He can often be found in the kitchen making my quick recipes.

At first, my husband was surprised by how much he enjoyed these healthier foods and that he didn't seem to miss his old favorites. What was most impressive to him was how much better he felt. He hadn't realized eating better and moving more could feel so good!

My husband now understood that he didn't have to be on a rigid diet—or any diet for that matter—to change his body composition and become stronger. As he began to exercise more, he became more aware that the number on the scale isn't a good indicator of his progress compared with measuring the inches around his waist.

He's thrilled with how he feels, his progress, and the ease of changing his ways much of the time (but not 100 percent of the time), and yet he's experiencing only the short-term effects. Given that he didn't go on a rigid, unforgiving plan that would be hard to continue throughout his life, he can continue to enjoy living a healthier lifestyle that weaves nicely into his busy life. He will live a stronger, better-quality life with fewer health issues, and I'll be right there with him enjoying the journey!

Transform Your Life For The Better

This is so much easier than you think and so much more enjoyable than you could imagine. You'll feel so much better, think better, and look better as you gain muscle, regardless of your present weight. Who doesn't want a better quality of life with more strength and fewer health issues?

Just start with one fix at a time!

Recipes For Success

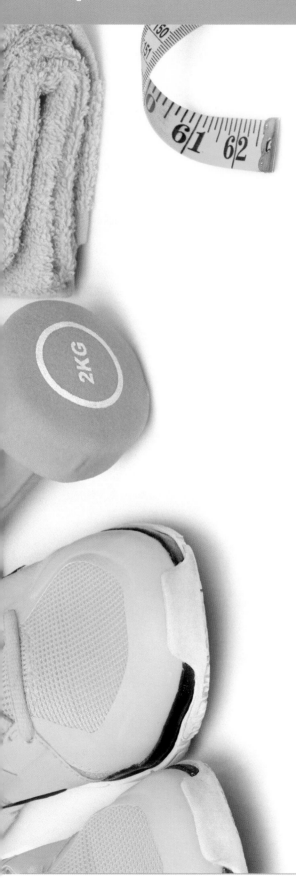

Throughout this book, I've shared some of my favorite recipes with you, but this is the one I love the most. It's my "recipe" for success. Using this 12-FIX LEAN LIFE PLAN recipe, you can improve your life and health by adding these special fix "ingredients" to your daily routine. Following this recipe will make you stronger and healthier than you've ever been.

Sometimes our lives become complicated. As with my other recipes, I've tried to simplify these ingredients and steps while still making the food we eat delicious and, in this case, effective. All twelve of these "ingredients" are important and should be observed when possible. However, adopting even one of these can benefit your health if you add it to your life's recipe most days from now on.

Prep time: Give yourself twelve weeks to add each ingredient to your life. Then give yourself twelve months to fully adopt the ingredients and steps in this recipe, and keep up the good work moving forward. By then, this will be a recipe you can make in your sleep.

Serves: 1 person—you!

Recipes Tips

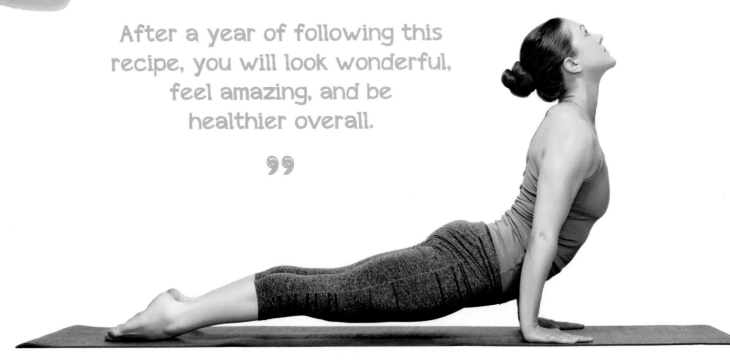

The biggest trick to following this recipe successfully is a positive attitude. There's no need to dwell on the times you miss an ingredient or don't act on a chosen behavior. Remember: this recipe is not an all-or-nothing endeavor.

In fact, the goal isn't to use all these ingredients 100 percent of the time. The goal is to use them most of the time, consistently for the rest of your life. After a year of following this recipe, you will look wonderful, feel amazing, and be healthier overall. You'll love the lifestyle and will want to follow it every day. You'll feel like you can conquer the world.

66

After a year of following this recipe, you will look wonderful, feel amazing, and be healthier overall.

99

Ingredients

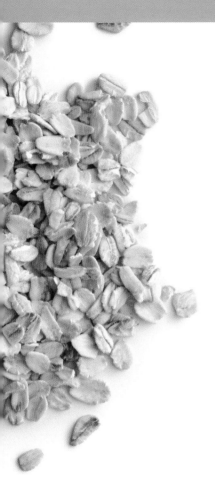

- **Fix #1:** Replace sugar, refined white flour, and processed foods with whole foods.

- **Fix #2:** Replace less-healthy fats with healthier fats.

- **Fix #3:** Eat a fermented food, like yogurt, every day.

- **Fix #4:** Rearrange your environment.

- **Fix #5:** Make fruits and vegetables 50% of your meals and snacks.

- **Fix #6:** Eat between three and six servings of whole grain per day.

- **Fix #7:** Front-load your eating.

- **Fix #8:** Chew small bites of food slowly and completely, eat only when you're hungry, and stop eating just before you get full.

- **Fix #9:** Drink water all day and evening.

- **Fix #10:** Eat a total of 75 to 150 grams protein spread out evenly through the day, with at least 30 grams of protein for breakfast.

- **Fix #11:** Move more.

- **Fix #12:** Sleep seven to eight hours every night.

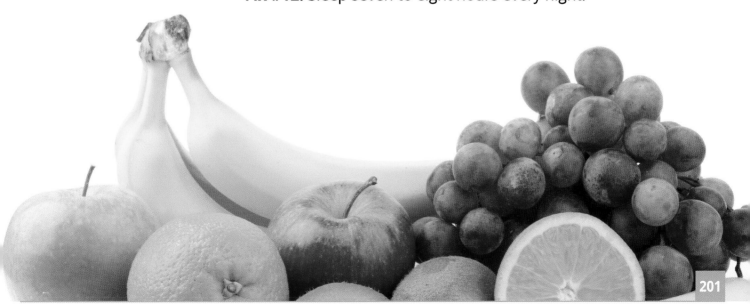

Directions

1. Begin by measuring your waist with a measuring tape. Take other body measurements too, if you wish. Write down these measurements and remeasure exactly the same way every month. If you have access to a body composition test, find out your body fat and lean tissue body percentages to begin and then retest every three months along with tracking your waist measurements. Don't be fooled by the number on a scale. This isn't a good indicator of the body fat you are losing. A gain in compact muscle (which you want) can mask the fat weight you lose, making it appear that you didn't lose as much body fat as you actually lost.

2. Add and focus on just one of these "fix" ingredients, one week at a time for twelve weeks. You can add them in any order you want; the recipe will succeed regardless, just as long as you add (not replace) one ingredient each week during your twelve-week jumpstart period. The LEAN BODY, SMART LIFE app will suggest the most advantageous fixes for you to start with to give you the best push forward.

3. Decide on your "focus fix" at the start of each week, along with some specific ways to make that change fit your lifestyle (see the action plans for each fix introduced throughout each of the previous chapters). Use the LEAN BODY, SMART LIFE app to track the fixes you add each week. Continue to follow and track the ones you already added.

4. After twelve weeks, you will have a chance to experience and track all twelve of these fix-ingredients. Continue following all twelve fixes but because it takes about thirty days to form a new habit, concentrate on ingraining the fixes you struggle with, one fix each month until all twelve fixes become an integral part of your life.

5. Make it a point to tell someone about your plan and the fix you have chosen to focus on. Encourage your friends and coworkers to try along with you. The LEAN BODY, SMART LIFE app allows you to share your progress with selected people, so you can support each other. You can even coordinate your "focus fix" to match each other. Let these friends, family, and coworkers be a means of accountability, and encourage each other to keep at it. Help one another to concentrate on the positive changes you're making, and don't forget to give each other a pat on the back to celebrate each small success!

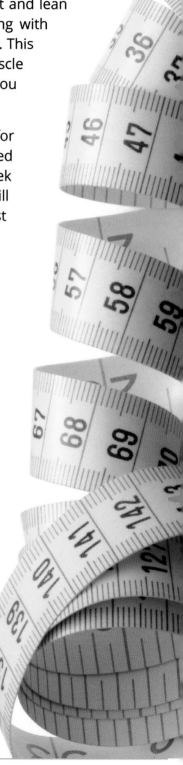

Serving It Up

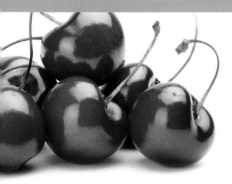

You've got this. This is the best recipe you can follow in your life, and you can do it!

In fact, some of the fixes in this recipe will be easier to adopt than you think—but they still need to be made into habits. Don't get stuck in the common and natural tendency to think that a fix is too small or too easy to really make a difference. Doing something, however small, is better than doing nothing. Remember that small changes over a long time make a bigger difference than lots of changes (hard or easy) over a short period of time.

So don't be discouraged if you are not perfect. You don't need to be perfect to succeed! Celebrate your successes instead of dwelling on failures. There are no failures in this recipe, except for giving up. Track the things you do right, not the things you do wrong, with the LEAN BODY, SMART LIFE app. Before you know it, guilt will vanish, and health and success will become a part of your everyday living.

The 12-FIX LEAN LIFE PLAN for a healthful, happy, and productive life is about feeling empowered by the health-promoting choices you make every day—even the little ones. Every fix you make, large or small, is going to have a positive impact on your well-being in the long run.

The ingredients are here, they're simple, and they're in your hands. Now that's a recipe for success for a smarter, healthier life!

 # Think About It

You don't have to be perfect with the fix you're focused on, but do try to be extremely mindful of it. Remember, the idea is to make a habit out of each ingredient you add. This will make it easier for you to turn each fix into the norm for the rest of your life, rather than being a temporary exception to the rule. That norm doesn't necessarily mean following a fix 100 percent of the time. That's the real point of this 12-FIX LEAN LIFE PLAN. Follow these fixes even 75 to 80 percent of the time for the rest of your life, and you will make a huge difference in your body composition, productivity, and your overall health.

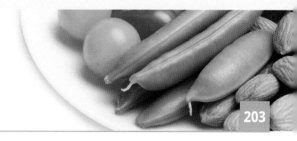

Bibliography

Intro chapter

- Huhn, Sebastian, Shahrzad Kharabian Masouleh, Michael Stumvoll, Arno Villringer, and A. Veronica Witte. "Components of a Mediterranean diet and their impact on cognitive functions in aging." Frontiers in Aging Neuroscience 7 (2015): 132.

- Centers for Disease Control and Prevention. "Chronic diseases: the power to prevent, the call to control. At a glance, 2009." Atlanta, GA: US Department of Health and Human Services (2009).

- Ludwig, David S., and Mark I. Friedman. "Increasing Adiposity: Consequences or Cause of Overeating?" JAMA 311, no. 21 (2014): 2167. doi:10.1001/jama.2014.4133.

- Carroll, Chrissy, MPH, RD. "Better Academic Performance—Is Nutrition the Missing Link?" Today's Dietitian, October 2014, 64.

- Ruscigno, Matthew, MPH, RD. "Brain Food for Older Adults." Today's Dietitian, June 2016, 22.

- Winer, Shawn, and Daniel A. Winer. "The adaptive immune system as a fundamental regulator of adipose tissue inflammation and insulin resistance." Immunology and Cell Biology 90, no. 8 (2012): 755-762.

- Cildir, Gökhan, Semih Can Akıncılar, and Vinay Tergaonkar. "Chronic adipose tissue inflammation: all immune cells on the stage." Trends in Molecular Medicine 19, no. 8 (2013): 487-500.

- Liebman, Bonnie. "Fighting Inflammation: It's Not as Simple as Some Claim." HighBeam Research - Newspaper archives and journal articles. November 1, 2011. Accessed April 27, 2017. https://www.highbeam.com/doc/1G1-271664924.html.

- Barbaresko, Janett, Manja Koch, Matthias B. Schulze, and Ute Nöthlings. "Dietary pattern analysis and biomarkers of low-grade inflammation: a systematic literature review." Nutrition Reviews 71, no. 8 (2013): 511-27. doi:10.1111/nure.12035.

- Galland, Leo. "Diet and Inflammation." Nutrition in Clinical Practice 25, no. 6 (2010): 634-40. doi:10.1177/0884533610385703.

- Zeyda, Maximilian, and Thomas M. Stulnig. "Obesity, Inflammation, and Insulin Resistance – A Mini-Review." Gerontology 55, no. 4 (2009): 379-86. doi:10.1159/000212758.

- Shivappa, Nitin, Susan E. Steck, Thomas G. Hurley, James R. Hussey, Yunsheng Ma, Ira S. Ockene, Fred Tabung, and James R. Hébert. "A population-based dietary inflammatory index predicts levels of C-reactive protein in the Seasonal Variation of Blood Cholesterol Study (SEASONS)." Public Health Nutrition 17, no. 08 (2013): 1825-833. doi:10.1017/s1368980013002565.

- Winer, Shawn, and Daniel A. Winer. "The adaptive immune system as a fundamental regulator of adipose tissue inflammation and insulin resistance." Immunology and Cell Biology 90, no. 8 (2012): 755-62. doi:10.1038/icb.2011.110.

- Glass, Christopher K., and Jerrold M. Olefsky. "Inflammation and Lipid Signaling in the Etiology of Insulin Resistance." Cell Metabolism 15, no. 5 (2012): 635-45. doi:10.1016/j.cmet.2012.04.001.

Chapter 1: Before Your Food

- "United States Department of Agriculture 2011 Dietary Guidelines for Americans ." Choose MyPlate. Accessed March 22, 2017. https://www.choosemyplate.gov/.

- Barclay, Eliza. "What Might Be Missing From MyPlate? Water." NPR. January 12, 2015. Accessed March 22, 2017. http://www.npr.org/sections/thesalt/2015/01/12/376172800/what-might-be-missing-from-myplate-water.

- Torbay, N., E. F. Bracco, A. Geliebter, I. M. Stewart, and S. A. Hashim. "Insulin increases body fat despite control of food intake and physical activity." American Journal of Physiology 248, no. 1 (January 1, 1985): R120-124.

- Ludwig DS, Friedman MI. Increasing adiposity: consequences or cause of overeating? JAMA 2014; 311(21);2167-2168

- Lumeng, C. N., and A. R. Saltiel. "Inflammatory links between obesity and metabolic disease." The Journal of Clinical Investigations 121, no. 6 (2011): 2111-117. doi:10.1172/JCI57132.

- Metter, E. Jeffrey, Laura A. Talbot, Matthew Schrager, and Robin Conwit. "Skeletal muscle strength as a predictor of all-cause mortality in healthy men." The Journals of Gerontology Series A: Biological Sciences and Medical Sciences 57, no. 10 (2002): B359-B365.

- Newman, Anne B., Varant Kupelian, Marjolein Visser, Eleanor M. Simonsick, Bret H. Goodpaster, Stephen B. Kritchevsky, Frances A. Tylavsky, Susan M. Rubin, and Tamara B. Harris. "Strength, but not muscle mass, is associated with mortality in the health, aging and body composition study cohort." The Journals of Gerontology Series A: Biological Sciences and Medical Sciences 61, no. 1 (2006): 72-77.

- Mozaffarian, Dariush, Tao Hao, Eric B. Rimm, Walter C. Willett, and Frank B. Hu. "Changes in Diet and Lifestyle and Long-Term Weight Gain in Women and Men." New England Journal of Medicine 364, no. 25 (June 23, 2011): 2392-404. doi:10.1056/nejmoa1014296.

Chapter 2: Know Your Food

- Liu, Rui Hai. "Health benefits of fruit and vegetables are from additive and synergistic combinations of phytochemicals." American Journal of Clinical Nutrition 78, no. 3 (September 2003): 517S-20S. http://ajcn.nutrition.org/content/78/3/517S.full.pdf html.

- Hung, H.-C., K. Joshipura, and W. Willett. "RESPONSE: Fruit and Vegetable Intake and Risk of Major Chronic Disease." Journal of the National Cancer Institute 96 (2004): 1577-584. doi:10.1093/jnci/dji107.

- Bhupathiraju, S. N., K. L. Tucker, and L. Katherine. "Greater variety in fruit and vegetable intake is associated with lower inflammation in Puerto Rican adults." American Journal of Clinical Nutrition 93, no. 1 (November 10, 2010): 37-46. doi:10.3945/ajcn.2010.29913.

- Bhupathiraju, S. N., N. M. Wedick, A. Pan, J. E. Manson, K. M. Rexrode, W. C. Willett, E. B. Rimm, and F. B. Hu. "Quantity and variety in fruit and vegetable intake and risk of coronary heart disease." American Journal of Clinical Nutrition 98, no. 6 (December 02, 2013): 1514-523. doi:10.3945/ajcn.113.066381.

- Boyer, Jeanelle, and Rui Hai Liu. "Apple phytochemicals and their health benefits." Nutrition Journal 3, no. 1 (May 12, 2004). doi:10.1186/1475-2891-3-5.

- Benton, David, Marie-Pierre Ruffin, Taous Lassel, Samantha Nabb, Michaël Messaoudi, Sophie Vinoy, Didier Desor, and Vincent Lang. "The delivery rate of dietary carbohydrates affects cognitive performance in both rats and humans." Psychopharmacology 166, no. 1 (2003): 86-90.

- Diano, Sabrina, Susan A. Farr, Stephen C. Benoit, Ewan C. McNay, Ivaldo da Silva, Balazs Horvath, F. Spencer Gaskin et al. "Ghrelin controls hippocampal spine synapse density and memory performance." Nature Neuroscience 9, no. 3 (2006): 381-388.

- Cao, Dongfeng, Hailin Lu, Terry L. Lewis, and Ling Li. "Intake of sucrose-sweetened water induces insulin resistance and exacerbates memory deficits and in a transgenic mouse model of Alzheimer disease." Journal of Biological Chemistry 282, no. 50 (2007): 36275-36282.

- Ahmed, Serge H., Karine Guillem, and Youna Vandaele. "Sugar addiction: pushing the drug-sugar analogy to the limit." Current Opinion in Clinical Nutrition and Metabolic Care 16, no. 4 (July 2013): 434-39. doi:10.1097/mco.0b013e328361c8b8.

- Lenoir, Magalie, Fuschia Serre, Lauriane Cantin, and Serge H. Ahmed. "Intense Sweetness Surpasses Cocaine Reward." PLoS One 2, no. 8 (August 01, 2007). doi:10.1371/journal.pone.0000698.

- Volkow, N. D., G. J. Wang, J. S. Fowler, D. Tomasi, and R. Baler. "Food and Drug Reward: Overlapping Circuits in Human Obesity and Addiction." Brain Imaging in Behavioral Neuroscience Current Topics in Behavioral Neurosciences, 20122, 1-24. doi:10.1007/7854_2011_169.

- Volkow, Nora D., Gene-Jack Wang, Dardo Tomasi, and Ruben D. Baler. "The Addictive Dimensionality of Obesity." Biological Psychiatry 73, no. 9 (May 1, 2013): 811-18. doi:10.1016/j.biopsych.2012.12.020.

- Hu, F. B. "Resolved: there is sufficient scientific evidence that decreasing sugar-sweetened beverage consumption will reduce the prevalence of obesity and obesity-related diseases." Obesity Reviews 14, no. 8 (August 13, 2013): 606-19. doi:10.1111/obr.12040.

- Wirfält, Elisabet, Isabel Drake, and Peter Wallström. "What do review papers conclude about food and dietary patterns?." Food & Nutrition Research 57 (2013).

- Mohapatra, D. P., V. Thakur, and S. K. Brar. "Antibacterial Efficacy of Raw and Processed Honey." Biotechnology Research International 2011 (2011): 1-6. doi:10.4061/2011/917505.

- Al-Waili, Noori S. "Natural Honey Lowers Plasma Glucose, C-Reactive Protein, Homocysteine, and Blood Lipids in Healthy, Diabetic, and Hyperlipidemic Subjects: Comparison with Dextrose and Sucrose." Journal of Medicinal Food 7, no. 1 (2004): 100-07. doi:10.1089/109662004322984789.

- Atkinson, Fiona S., Kaye Foster-Powell, and Jennie C. Brand-Miller. "International tables of glycemic index and glycemic load values: 2008." Diabetes Care 31, no. 12 (2008): 2281-2283.

- Drake, R., D. Felbaum, C. Huntley, A. Reed, L. Matthews, and B. Raudenbush. "Effects of chocolate consumption on enhancing cognitive performance." Appetite 49, no. 1 (2007): 288.

- Jonnalagadda, S. S., L. Harnack, R. Hai Liu, N. Mckeown, C. Seal, S. Liu, and G. C. Fahey. "Putting the Whole Grain Puzzle Together: Health Benefits Associated with Whole Grains--Summary of American Society for Nutrition 2010 Satellite Symposium." Journal of Nutrition 141, no. 5 (March 30, 2011). doi:10.3945/jn.110.132944.

- Specter, Michael. "What's So Bad About Gluten?" The New Yorker. October 26, 2014. Accessed March 23, 2017. http://www.newyorker.com/magazine/2014/11/03/grain.

- Gibson, Peter R., and Susan J. Shepherd. "Evidence□based dietary management of functional gastrointestinal symptoms: The FODMAP approach." Journal of Gastroenterology and Hepatology 25, no. 2 (2010): 252-258.

- Nanda, Rakesh, Lin H. Shu, and J. Reggie Thomas. "A FODMAP Diet Update: Craze or Credible?." Practical Gastroenterology (2012): 37.

- Granholm, Ann-Charlotte, Heather A. Bimonte-Nelson, Alfred B. Moore, Matthew E. Nelson, Linnea R. Freeman, and Kumar Sambamurti. "Effects of a saturated fat and high cholesterol diet on memory and hippocampal morphology in the middle-aged rat." Journal of Alzheimer's Disease 14, no. 2 (2008): 133-145.

- Weisenberger, Jill, MS, RDN, CDE. "The Omega Fats." Today's Dietitian, April 2014, 20.

- Titos, Esther, and Joan Clària. "Omega-3-derived mediators counteract obesity-induced adipose tissue inflammation." Prostaglandins & Other Lipid Mediators 107 (2013): 77-84.

- Calder, Philip C. "Omega-3 fatty acids and inflammatory processes." Nutrients 2, no. 3 (2010): 355-374.

- Gardener, Samantha L., Stephanie R. Rainey-Smith, M. B. Barnes, Hamid R. Sohrabi, M. Weinborn, Yen Ying Lim, Karra Harrington et al. "Dietary patterns and cognitive decline in an Australian study of ageing." Molecular Psychiatry 20, no. 7 (2015): 860-866.

- Bradbury, Joanne. "Docosahexaenoic acid (DHA): an ancient nutrient for the modern human brain." Nutrients 3, no. 5 (2011): 529-554.

- Harrar, Sari. "Omega-3 Fatty Acids and Mood Disorders." Today's Dietitian, January 2012, 22.

- Sarris, Jerome, David Mischoulon, and Isaac Schweitzer. "Omega-3 for bipolar disorder: meta-analyses of use in mania and bipolar depression." (2012): 81-86.

- Tone, Clare, MS, RD. "Omegas: Omega-3 Fats and Pregnancy — Health Benefits for Both Mom and Baby." Today's Dietitian, May 2016, 14.

- Hibbeln, Joseph R. "Seafood consumption, the DHA content of mothers' milk and prevalence rates of postpartum depression: a cross-national, ecological analysis." Journal of Affective Disorders 69, no. 1 (2002): 15-29.

- Weisenberger, Jill. "Heart-Healthy Fats — It's the Type—Not the Amount—That Matters." Today's Dietitian, September 2013, 14.

- Schwingshackl, L., B. Strasser, and G. Hoffmann. "Effects of monounsaturated fatty acids on cardiovascular risk factors: a systematic review and meta-analysis." Annals of Nutrition and Metabolism 59, no. 2-4 (2011): 176-186.

- Liu, Xiaoran, Penny M. Kris-Etherton, Sheila G. West, Benoît Lamarche, David J.a. Jenkins, Jennifer A. Fleming, Cindy E. Mccrea, Shuaihua Pu, Patrick Couture, Philip W. Connelly, and Peter J.h. Jones. "Effects of canola and high-oleic-acid canola oils on abdominal fat mass in individuals with central obesity." Obesity 24, no. 11 (November 2016): 2261-268. doi:10.1002/oby.21584.

- Gillingham, Leah G., Sydney Harris-Janz, and Peter JH Jones. "Dietary monounsaturated fatty acids are protective against metabolic syndrome and cardiovascular disease risk factors." Lipids 46, no. 3 (2011): 209-228.

- van Dijk, Susan J., Edith JM Feskens, Marieke B. Bos, Lisette CPGM de Groot, Jeanne HM de Vries, Michael Müller, and Lydia A. Afman. "Consumption of a high monounsaturated fat diet reduces oxidative phosphorylation gene expression in peripheral blood mononuclear cells of abdominally overweight men and women." The Journal of Nutrition 142, no. 7 (2012): 1219-1225.

- Lin, Lin, Hanja Allemekinders, Angela Dansby, Lisa Campbell, Shaunda Durance-Tod, Alvin Berger, and Peter JH Jones. "Evidence of health benefits of canola oil." Nutrition Reviews 71, no. 6 (2013): 370-385.

- Jones, Peter JH, Dylan S. MacKay, Vijitha K. Senanayake, Shuaihua Pu, David JA Jenkins, Philip W. Connelly, Benoît Lamarche et al. "High-oleic canola oil consumption enriches LDL particle cholesteryl oleate content and reduces LDL proteoglycan binding in humans." Atherosclerosis 238, no. 2 (2015): 231-238

- McCulloch, Marsha, MS, RD, LD. "Saturated Fat: Not So Bad or Just Bad Science?" Today's Dietitian, November 2014, 32.

- Brehm, Bonnie J., and David A. D'alessio. "Benefits of high-protein weight loss diets: enough evidence for practice?" Current Opinion in Endocrinology, Diabetes and Obesity 15, no. 5 (October 2008): 416-21. doi:10.1097/med.0b013e328308dc13.

- Paddon-Jones, D., E. Westman, R. D. Mattes, R. R. Wolfe, A. Astrup, and M. Westerterp-Plantenga. "Protein, weight management, and satiety." American Journal of Clinical Nutrition 87, no. 5 (May 2008): 1558S-561S.

- Paddon-Jones, D., K. R. Short, W. W. Campbell, E. Volpi, and R. R. Wolfe. "Role of dietary protein in the sarcopenia of aging." American Journal of Clinical Nutrition 87, no. 5 (May 2008): 1562S-1566S.

- Welland, Diane. "Lose Weight the High-Protein Weigh." Today's Dietitian, February 2010, 34.

- Mcguire, S. "U.S. Department of Agriculture and U.S. Department of Health and Human Services, Dietary Guidelines for Americans, 2010. 7th Edition, Washington, DC: U.S. Government Printing Office, January 2011." Advances in Nutrition: An International Review Journal 2, no. 3 (December 01, 2010): 293-94. doi:10.3945/an.111.000430.

- O'Connor, Laura M., Marleen A. H. Lentjes, Robert N. Luben, Kay-Tee Khaw, Nicholas J. Wareham, and Nita G. Forouhi. "Dietary dairy product intake and incident type 2 diabetes: a prospective study using dietary data from a 7-day food diary." Diabetologia 57, no. 5 (May 08, 2014): 909-17. doi:10.1007/s00125-014-3176-1.

- Wang, Huifen, Kara A. Livingston, Caroline S. Fox, James B. Meigs, and Paul F. Jacques. "Yogurt consumption is associated with better diet quality and metabolic profile in American men and women." Nutrition Research 33, no. 1 (January 2013): 18-26. doi:10.1016/j.nutres.2012.11.009.

- Ralston, N. Selenium: The Secret That Will Change Public Perception of Seafood. Talk presented at: Academy of Nutrition and Dietetics 2016 Food and Nutrition Conference & Expo; October 16, 2016; Boston, MA.

- Ralston, NV and Raymond, NJ. (November 2010). Dietary selenium's protective effects against methylmercury toxicity. Toxicology, 278(1).

- U.S. Food and Drug Administration. (June 2014). Fish: What Pregnant Women and Parents Should Know. Draft Updated Advice by FDA and EPA.

- Mozaffarian, Dariush, Tao Hao, Eric B. Rimm, Walter C. Willett, and Frank B. Hu. "Changes in Diet and Lifestyle and Long-Term Weight Gain in Women and Men." New England Journal of Medicine 364, no. 25 (2011): 2392-404. doi:10.1056/nejmoa1014296.

- Bonjour, Jean-Philippe. "Dietary Protein: An Essential Nutrient For Bone Health." Journal of the American College of Nutrition 24, no. 6 (December 2005). 10.1080/07315724.2005.10719501.

- Everard, Amandine, and Patrice D. Cani. "Diabetes, obesity and gut microbiota." Best Practice & Research Clinical Gastroenterology 27, no. 1 (2013): 73-83.

- Zanteson, Lori. "Gut Health and Immunity — It's All About the Good Bacteria That Can Help Fight Disease." Today's Dietitian, June 2012, 58.

- Wang, Wei-Lin, Shao-Yan Xu, Zhi-Gang Ren, Liang Tao, Jian-Wen Jiang, and Shu-Sen Zheng. "Application of metagenomics in the human gut microbiome." World Journal of Gastroenterology: WJG 21, no. 3 (2015): 803.

- Ding, Shengli, and Pauline K. Lund. "Role of intestinal inflammation as an early event in obesity and insulin resistance." Current Opinion in Clinical Nutrition and Metabolic Care 14, no. 4 (2011): 328.

- Caricilli, Andrea M., and Mario JA Saad. "The role of gut microbiota on insulin resistance." Nutrients 5, no. 3 (2013): 829-851.

- Lam, Yan Y., Andrew J. Mitchell, Andrew J. Holmes, Gareth S. Denyer, Anders Gummesson, Ian D. Caterson, Nicholas H. Hunt, and Len H. Storlien. "Role of the gut in visceral fat inflammation and metabolic disorders." Obesity 19, no. 11 (2011): 2113-2120.

- Getz, Lindsey. "A Healthful Dose of Bacteria — Yogurt Is the Best Probiotic Source, but Clients Do Have Other Options." Today's Dietitian, October 2011, 46.

- Schaeffer, Juliann. "Dairy's Probiotic Power — A Review of the Benefits of Probiotics, the Top Sources, and What's New in the Dairy Case." Today's Dietitian, August 2014, 32.

- Bengmark, Stig. "Gut microbiota, immune development and function." Pharmacological Research 69, no. 1 (March 2013): 87-113. doi:10.1016/j.phrs.2012.09.002.

- Brown-Riggs, Constance, MSEd, RD, CDE, CDN. "The Gut Microbiota — Is It a Novel Contributor to the Obesity and Diabetes Epidemics?" Today's Dietitian, November 2014, 22.

- Baumler, Megan D., PhD, RD, CD. "Gut Bacteria." Today's Dietitian, June 2013, 46.

- Pearson, Helen. "Fat people harbour 'fat' microbes." Nature, December 18, 2006. doi:10.1038/news061218-6.

- Selhub, Eva M., Alan C. Logan, and Alison C. Bested. "Fermented foods, microbiota, and mental health: ancient practice meets nutritional psychiatry." Journal of Physiological Anthropology 33, no. 1 (January 15, 2014): 2. doi:10.1186/1880-6805-33-2.

- Brahe, L. K., A. Astrup, and L. H. Larsen. "Is butyrate the link between diet, intestinal microbiota and obesity-related metabolic diseases?" Obesity Reviews 14, no. 12 (December 16, 2013): 950-59. doi:10.1111/obr.12068.

- Lombardo, Nancy Emerson. "Nutrition's Potency to Help or Hurt Brain Health & Our Challenge." Proceedings of Food & Nutrition Conference & Expo 2016, Boston Convention and Exhibition Center, Boston.

- Holscher, Hannah. "The Gut-Brain Highway: Can Traffic Be Regulated by Diet?" Proceedings of Food & Nutrition Conference & Expo 2016, Boston Convention and Exhibition Center, Boston.

- Carabotti, Marilia, Annunziata Scirocco, Maria Antonietta Maselli, and Carola Severi. "The gut-brain axis: interactions between enteric microbiota, central and enteric nervous systems." Annals of Gastroenterology: Quarterly Publication of the Hellenic Society of Gastroenterology 28, no. 2 (2015): 203.

- Mayer, Emeran A., Rob Knight, Sarkis K. Mazmanian, John F. Cryan, and Kirsten Tillisch. "Gut microbes and the brain: paradigm shift in neuroscience." Journal of Neuroscience 34, no. 46 (2014): 15490-15496.

- Foster, Jane A., Mark Lyte, Emeran Meyer, and John F. Cryan. "Gut microbiota and brain function: an evolving field in neuroscience." International Journal of Neuropsychopharmacology 19, no. 5 (2016): pyv114.

- Collins, Sherry Coleman, MS, RDN, LD. "Entering the World of Prebiotics — Are They a Precursor to Good Gut Health?" Today's Dietitian, December 2014, 12.

- Sun, Jiadong, Hang Ma, Navindra P. Seeram, and David C. Rowley. "Detection of Inulin, a Prebiotic Polysaccharide, in Maple Syrup." Journal of Agricultural and Food Chemistry 64, no. 38 (2016): 7142-7147.

Chapter 3: Eat Your Food

- Watkins, Julia A. "Mindless Eating: Why We Eat More Than We Think, Brian Wansink, Ph.D." The Journal of Behavioral Health Services & Research 35, no. 2 (January 16, 2008): 235-36. doi:10.1007/s11414-007-9102-2.

- Robinson, Eric. "Slim by Design: Mindless Eating Solutions for Everyday Life. By Brian Wansink. William Morrow & Company: New York, 2014." Obesity Reviews 16, no. 2 (January 23, 2015): 187-88. doi:10.1111/obr.12249.

- Wansink, B., J. E. Painter, and Y-K Lee. "The office candy dish: proximity's influence on estimated and actual consumption." International Journal of Obesity 30, no. 5 (2006): 871-75. doi:10.1038/sj.ijo.0803217.

- Wansink, Brian, James E. Painter, and Jill North. "Bottomless Bowls: Why Visual Cues of Portion Size May Influence Intake." Obesity Research 13, no. 1 (January 2005): 93-100. doi:10.1038/oby.2005.12.

- Wansink, Brian, and Matthew M. Cheney. "Super Bowls: Serving Bowl Size and Food Consumption." JAMA 293, no. 14 (April 13, 2005): 1727-728. doi:10.1001/jama.293.14.1727.

- Wansink, Brian, and Junyong Kim. "Bad Popcorn in Big Buckets: Portion Size Can Influence Intake as Much as Taste." Journal of Nutrition Education and Behavior 37, no. 5 (Sept. & oct. 2005): 242-45. doi:10.1016/s1499-4046(06)60278-9.

- Wansink, B., and Koert Van Ittersum. "Shape of glass and amount of alcohol poured: comparative study of effect of practice and concentration." BMJ 331, no. 7531 (December 24, 2005): 1512-514. doi:10.1136/bmj.331.7531.1512.

Chapter 4: Track Your Food

- Hollis, James, and Richard Mattes. "Effect of chronic consumption of almonds on body weight in healthy humans." British Journal of Nutrition 98, no. 03 (September 20, 2007): 651-56. doi:10.1017/s0007114507734608.

- Wien, M. A., J. M. Sabaté, D. N. Iklé, and F. R. Kandeel. "Almonds vs complex carbohydrates in a weight reduction program." International Journal of Obesity 27, no. 11 (November 2004): 1365-372. doi:10.1038/sj.ijo.0802411.

- Mattes, R.D., and M. L. Dreher. "Nuts and healthy body weight maintenance mechanisms." Asia Pac. J. Clin. Nutr. 19, no. 1 (2010): 137-41.

- Mattes, R.D. "The energetics of nut consumption." Asia Pac. J. Clin. Nutr. 17, no. S1 (2008): 337-39.

- Rajaram, Sujatha, and Joan Sabaté. "Nuts, body weight and insulin resistance." British Journal of Nutrition 96, no. S2 (November 2006): S79-86. doi:10.1017/bjn20061867.

- Jaceldo-Siegl, Karen, Joan Sabaté, Sujatha Rajaram, and Gary E. Fraser. "Long-term almond supplementation without advice on food replacement induces favourable nutrient modifications to the habitual diets of free-living individuals." British Journal of Nutrition 92, no. 03 (September 2004): 533-40. doi:10.1079/bjn20041223.

- Fraser, Gary E., Hannelore W. Bennett, Karen B. Jaceldo, and Joan Sabaté. "Effect on Body Weight of a Free 76 Kilojoule (320 Calorie) Daily Supplement of Almonds for Six Months." Journal of the American College of Nutrition 21, no. 3 (June 2002): 275-83. doi:10.1080/07315724.2002.10719221.

- Tan, S. Y., and R. D. Mattes. "Appetitive, dietary and health effects of almonds consumed with meals or as snacks: a randomized, controlled trial." European Journal of Clinical Nutrition 67, no. 11 (October 02, 2013): 1205-214. doi:10.1038/ejcn.2013.184.

- California, Almond Board of. "Are Almonds An Optimal Snack?" PR Newswire: news distribution, targeting and monitoring. April 25, 2014. Accessed April 25, 2017. http://www.prnewswire.com/news-releases/are-almonds-an-optimal-snack-256680241.html.

- Hollis, Jack F., Christina M. Gullion, Victor J. Stevens, Phillip J. Brantley, Lawrence J. Appel, Jamy D. Ard, Catherine M. Champagne, Arlene Dalcin, Thomas P. Erlinger, Kristine Funk, Daniel Laferriere, Pao-Hwa Lin, Catherine M. Loria, Carmen Samuel-Hodge, William M. Vollmer, and Laura P. Svetkey. "Weight Loss During the Intensive Intervention Phase of the Weight-Loss Maintenance Trial." American Journal of Preventive Medicine 35, no. 2 (August 2008): 118-26. doi:10.1016/j.amepre.2008.04.013.

- Kaiser Permanente. Press Release. "Kaiser Permanente Study Finds Keeping a Food Diary Doubles Diet Weight Loss." News release, July 8, 2008. Kaiserpermanente.org. https://share.kaiserpermanente.org/article/kaiser-permanente-study-finds-keeping-a-food-diary-doubles-diet-weight-loss/.

- Ebbeling, Cara B., Janis F. Swain, Henry A. Feldman, William W. Wong, David L. Hachey, Erica Garcia-Lago, and David S. Ludwig. "Effects of Dietary Composition During Weight Loss Maintenance: A Controlled Feeding Study." JAMA: Journal of the American Medical Association 307, no. 24 (2012): 2627.

- Lampe, J. W. "Health effects of vegetables and fruit: assessing mechanisms of action in human experimental studies." American Journal of Clinical Nutrition 70, no. 3 (September 1999): 475S-90S. http://www.ncbi.nlm.nih.gov/pubmed/10479220.

- Shivappa, N., S. E. Steck, T. G. Hurley, J. R. Hussey, Y. Ma, I. S. Ockene, F. Tabung, and J. R. Hebert. "A population-based dietary inflammatory index predicts levels of C-reactive protein in the Seasonal Variation of Blood Cholesterol Study (SEASONS)." Public Health Nutrition 17, no. 8 (August 2014): 1825-833. doi: 10.1017/S1368980013002565.

- Shivappa, Nitin. "Dietary Inflammatory Index and its relationship with inflammation, metabolic biomarkers and mortality." (2014).

- Aune, Dagfinn, Edward Giovannucci, Paolo Boffetta, Lars T. Fadnes, NaNa Keum, Teresa Norat, Darren C. Greenwood, Elio Riboli, Lars J. Vatten, and Serena Tonstad. "Fruit and vegetable intake and the risk of cardiovascular disease, total cancer and all-cause mortality–a systematic review and dose-response meta-analysis of prospective studies." International Journal of Epidemiology (2017): dyw319.

- Zandi, Peter P., James C. Anthony, Ara S. Khachaturian, Stephanie V. Stone, Deborah Gustafson, JoAnn T. Tschanz, Maria C. Norton, Kathleen A. Welsh-Bohmer, and John CS Breitner. "Reduced risk of Alzheimer disease in users of antioxidant vitamin supplements: the Cache County Study." Archives of Neurology 61, no. 1 (2004): 82-88.

- "Link between vitamin A and learning abilities established by team led by Salk researchers." Salk Institute for Biological Studies. December 22, 1998. Accessed April 25, 2017. http://www.salk.edu/news/pressrelease_details.php?press_id=50.

- Polidori, M. Cristina, Domenico Praticó, Francesca Mangialasche, Elena Mariani, Olivier Aust, Timur Anlasik, Ni Mang et al. "High fruit and vegetable intake is positively correlated with antioxidant status and cognitive performance in healthy subjects." Journal of Alzheimer's Disease 17, no. 4 (2009): 921-927.

- Martin, A., A. Cherubini, C. Andres-Lacueva, M. Paniagua, and J. Joseph. "Effects of fruits and vegetables on levels of vitamins E and C in the brain and their association with cognitive performance." The Journal of Nutrition, Health & Aging 6, no. 6 (2001): 392-404.

- Polidori, M. Cristina, Domenico Praticó, Francesca Mangialasche, Elena Mariani, Olivier Aust, Timur Anlasik, Ni Mang et al. "High fruit and vegetable intake is positively correlated with antioxidant status and cognitive performance in healthy subjects." Journal of Alzheimer's Disease 17, no. 4 (2009): 921-927.

- Florence, Michelle D., Mark Asbridge, and Paul J. Veugelers. "Diet quality and academic performance." Journal of School Health 78, no. 4 (2008): 209-215.

- Martin, A., A. Cherubini, C. Andres-Lacueva, M. Paniagua, and J. Joseph. "Effects of fruits and vegetables on levels of vitamins E and C in the brain and their association with cognitive performance." The Journal of Nutrition, Health & Aging 6, no. 6 (2001): 392-404.

- Desjardins, Yves. "Fruit and vegetables and health: an overview." In Horticulture: Plants for People and Places, Volume 3, pp. 965-1000. Springer Netherlands, 2014.

- Whyte, Adrian R., Graham Schafer, and Claire M. Williams. "Cognitive effects following acute wild blueberry supplementation in 7-to 10-year-old children." European Journal of Nutrition 55, no. 6 (2016): 2151-2162.

- Miller, Marshall G., and Barbara Shukitt-Hale. "Berry fruit enhances beneficial signaling in the brain." Journal of Agricultural and Food Chemistry 60, no. 23 (2012): 5709-5715.

- Layman, Donald K. "Dietary Guidelines should reflect new understandings about adult protein needs." Nutrition & Metabolism 6, no. 1 (2009): 12.

- Brown, Lisa, Bernard Rosner, Walter W. Willett, and Frank M. Sacks. "Cholesterol-lowering effects of dietary fiber: a meta-analysis." The American Journal of Clinical Nutrition 69, no. 1 (1999): 30-42.

- Olga, Cernelev. "A Survey On Dietary Intake And Eating Habits Among The Students From The Republic Of Moldova." Global Journal of Multidisciplinary Studies 5, no. 11 (2016).

- Ozawa, Mio, Martin Shipley, Mika Kivimaki, Archana Singh-Manoux, and Eric J. Brunner. "Dietary pattern, inflammation and cognitive decline: The Whitehall II prospective cohort study." Clinical Nutrition 36, no. 2 (2017): 506-512.

- Carroll, Chrissy, MPH, RD. "Better Academic Performance — Is Nutrition the Missing Link?" Today's Dietitian, October 2014, 64.

Chapter 5: Time Your Food

- Leidy, Heather J., Laura C. Ortinau, Steve M. Douglas, and Heather A. Hoertel. "Beneficial effects of a higher-protein breakfast on the appetitive, hormonal, and neural signals controlling energy intake regulation in overweight/obese,"breakfast-skipping," late-adolescent girls." The American Journal of Clinical Nutrition 97, no. 4 (2013): 677-688.

- Leidy, Heather J., Mandi J. Bossingham, Richard D. Mattes, and Wayne W. Campbell. "Increased dietary protein consumed at breakfast leads to an initial and sustained feeling of fullness during energy restriction compared to other meal times." British Journal of Nutrition 101, no. 06 (2009): 798-803.

- Leidy, H. J., and E. M. Racki. "The addition of a protein-rich breakfast and its effects on acute appetite control and food intake in 'breakfast-skipping' adolescents." International Journal of Obesity 34, no. 7 (2010): 1125-1133.

- Vander Wal, J. S., A. Gupta, P. Khosla, and N. V. Dhurandhar. "Egg breakfast enhances weight loss." International Journal of Obesity 32, no. 10 (2008): 1545-1551.

- Zeisel, Steven H., and Kerry-Ann Da Costa. "Choline: an essential nutrient for public health." Nutrition Reviews 67, no. 11 (2009): 615-623.

- Garaulet, Marta, Purificación Gómez-Abellán, Juan J. Alburquerque-Béjar, Yu-Chi Lee, Jose M. Ordovás, and Frank AJL Scheer. "Timing of food intake predicts weight loss effectiveness." International Journal of Obesity 37, no. 4 (2013): 604-611.

- Jakubowicz, Daniela, Maayan Barnea, Julio Wainstein, and Oren Froy. "High caloric intake at breakfast vs. dinner differentially influences weight loss of overweight and obese women." Obesity 21, no. 12 (2013): 2504-2512.

- Bo, Simona, Giovanni Musso, Guglielmo Beccuti, Maurizio Fadda, Debora Fedele, Roberto Gambino, Luigi Gentile, Marilena Durazzo, Ezio Ghigo, and Maurizio Cassader. "Consuming more of daily caloric intake at dinner predisposes to obesity. A 6-year population-based prospective cohort study." PloS One 9, no. 9 (2014): e108467.

- Oike, Hideaki, Katsutaka Oishi, and Masuko Kobori. "Nutrients, clock genes, and chrononutrition." Current Nutrition Reports 3, no. 3 (2014): 204-212.

- Jakubowicz, Daniela, Oren Froy, Julio Wainstein, and Mona Boaz. "Meal timing and composition influence ghrelin levels, appetite scores and weight loss maintenance in overweight and obese adults." Steroids 77, no. 4 (2012): 323-331.

- Vollmers, Christopher, Shubhroz Gill, Luciano DiTacchio, Sandhya R. Pulivarthy, Hiep D. Le, and Satchidananda Panda. "Time of feeding and the intrinsic circadian clock drive rhythms in hepatic gene expression." Proceedings of the National Academy of Sciences 106, no. 50 (2009): 21453-21458.

- Cho, Han, Xuan Zhao, Megumi Hatori, T. Yu Ruth, Grant D. Barish, Michael T. Lam, Ling-Wa Chong et al. "Regulation of circadian behaviour and metabolism by REV-ERB-[agr] and REV-ERB-[bgr]." Nature 485, no. 7396 (2012): 123-127.

- Wansink, Brian, Collin R. Payne, and Pierre Chandon. "Internal and external cues of meal cessation: The French paradox redux?." Obesity 15, no. 12 (2007): 2920-2924.

- Andrade, Ana M., Geoffrey W. Greene, and Kathleen J. Melanson. "Eating slowly led to decreases in energy intake within meals in healthy women." Journal of the American Dietetic Association 108, no. 7 (2008): 1186-1191.

- Li, Jie, Na Zhang, Lizhen Hu, Ze Li, Rui Li, Cong Li, and Shuran Wang. "Improvement in chewing activity reduces energy intake in one meal and modulates plasma gut hormone concentrations in obese and lean young Chinese men." The American Journal of Clinical Nutrition 94, no. 3 (2011): 709-716.

Chapter 6: Burn Your Food

- Ebbeling, Cara B., Janis F. Swain, Henry A. Feldman, William W. Wong, David L. Hachey, Erica Garcia-Lago, and David S. Ludwig. "Effects of dietary composition on energy expenditure during weight-loss maintenance." JAMA 307, no. 24 (2012): 2627-2634.

- Pourhassan, Maryam, Anja Bosy-Westphal, Britta Schautz, Wiebke Braun, Claus-C. Glüer, and Manfred J. Müller. "Impact of body composition during weight change on resting energy expenditure and homeostasis model assessment index in overweight nonsmoking adults." The American Journal of Clinical Nutrition (2014): ajcn-071829.

- Schwartz, A., and E. Doucet. "Relative changes in resting energy expenditure during weight loss: a systematic review." Obesity Reviews 11, no. 7 (2010): 531-547.

- Weigle, David S., Karon J. Sande, Per-Henrik Iverius, Elaine R. Monsen, and John D. Brunzell. "Weight loss leads to a marked decrease in nonresting energy expenditure in ambulatory human subjects." Metabolism 37, no. 10 (1988): 930-936.

- Spieth, Leslie E., Jennifer D. Harnish, Carine M. Lenders, Lauren B. Raezer, Mark A. Pereira, S. Jan Hangen, and David S. Ludwig. "A low–glycemic index diet in the treatment of pediatric obesity." Archives of Pediatrics & Adolescent Medicine 154, no. 9 (2000): 947-951.

- Ludwig, David S., Joseph A. Majzoub, Ahmad Al-Zahrani, Gerard E. Dallal, Isaac Blanco, and Susan B. Roberts. "High glycemic index foods, overeating, and obesity." Pediatrics 103, no. 3 (1999): e26-e26.

- Chandler-Laney, Paula C., Shannon A. Morrison, Laura Lee T. Goree, Amy C. Ellis, Krista Casazza, Renee Desmond, and Barbara A. Gower. "Return of hunger following a relatively high carbohydrate breakfast is associated with earlier recorded glucose peak and nadir." Appetite 80 (2014): 236-241.

- Raben, Anne, Lisa Agerholm-Larsen, Anne Flint, Jens J. Holst, and Arne Astrup. "Meals with similar energy densities but rich in protein, fat, carbohydrate, or alcohol have different effects on energy expenditure and substrate metabolism but not on appetite and energy intake." The American Journal of Clinical Nutrition 77, no. 1 (2003): 91-100.

- Soenen, Stijn, and Margriet S. Westerterp-Plantenga. "Proteins and satiety: implications for weight management." Current Opinion in Clinical Nutrition & Metabolic Care 11, no. 6 (2008): 747-751.

- Layman, Donald K., Richard A. Boileau, Donna J. Erickson, James E. Painter, Harn Shiue, Carl Sather, and Demtra D. Christou. "A reduced ratio of dietary carbohydrate to protein improves body composition and blood lipid profiles during weight loss in adult women." The Journal of Nutrition 133, no. 2 (2003): 411-417.

- Barr, SadieB, and JonathanC Wright. "Postprandial energy expenditure in whole-food and processed-food meals: implications for daily energy expenditure." Food & Nutrition Research 54, no. 1 (2010): 5144.

- Karl, J. Philip, Mohsen Meydani, Junaidah B. Barnett, Sally M. Vanegas, Barry Goldin, Anne Kane, Helen Rasmussen et al. "Substituting whole grains for refined grains in a 6-wk randomized trial favorably affects energy-balance metrics in healthy men and postmenopausal women." The American Journal of Clinical Nutrition 105, no. 3 (2017): 589-599.

- Mozaffarian, Dariush, Tao Hao, Eric B. Rimm, Walter C. Willett, and Frank B. Hu. "Changes in Diet and Lifestyle and Long-Term Weight Gain in Women and Men." New England Journal of Medicine 364, no. 25 (June 23, 2011): 2392-404. doi:10.1056/nejmoa1014296.

- Bes-Rastrollo, Maira, Nicole M. Wedick, Miguel Angel Martinez-Gonzalez, Tricia Y. Li, Laura Sampson, and Frank B. Hu. "Prospective study of nut consumption, long-term weight change, and obesity risk in women." The American Journal of Clinical Nutrition 89, no. 6 (2009): 1913-1919.

- Traoret, C. J., P. Lokko, A. C. R. F. Cruz, C. G. Oliveira, N. M. B. Costa, J. Bressan, R. C. G. Alfenas, and R. D. Mattes. "Peanut digestion and energy balance." International Journal of Obesity 32, no. 2 (2008): 322-328.

- Vanegas, Sally M., Mohsen Meydani, Junaidah B. Barnett, Barry Goldin, Anne Kane, Helen Rasmussen, Carrie Brown et al. "Substituting whole grains for refined grains in a 6-wk randomized trial has a modest effect on gut microbiota and immune and inflammatory markers of healthy adults." The American Journal of Clinical Nutrition 105, no. 3 (2017): 635-650.

- Krajmalnik-Brown, Rosa, Zehra-Esra Ilhan, Dae-Wook Kang, and John K. DiBaise. "Effects of gut microbes on nutrient absorption and energy regulation." Nutrition in Clinical Practice 27, no. 2 (2012): 201-214.

- Stookey, Jodi D., Florence Constant, Christopher D. Gardner, and Barry M. Popkin. "Replacing sweetened caloric beverages with drinking water is associated with lower energy intake." Obesity 15, no. 12 (2007): 3013-3022.

- Mattes, Richard D. "Hunger and thirst: issues in measurement and prediction of eating and drinking." Physiology & Behavior 100, no. 1 (2010): 22-32.

- Boschmann, Michael, Jochen Steiniger, Uta Hille, Jens Tank, Frauke Adams, Arya M. Sharma, Susanne Klaus, Friedrich C. Luft, and Jens Jordan. "Water-induced thermogenesis." The Journal of Clinical Endocrinology & Metabolism 88, no. 12 (2003): 6015-6019.

- Schulze, Matthias B., JoAnn E. Manson, David S. Ludwig, Graham A. Colditz, Meir J. Stampfer, Walter C. Willett, and Frank B. Hu. "Sugar-sweetened beverages, weight gain, and incidence of type 2 diabetes in young and middle-aged women." JAMA 292, no. 8 (2004): 927-934.

- Armstrong, Lawrence E., Matthew S. Ganio, Douglas J. Casa, Elaine C. Lee, Brendon P. McDermott, Jennifer F. Klau, Liliana Jimenez, Laurent Le Bellego, Emmanuel Chevillotte, and Harris R. Lieberman. "Mild dehydration affects mood in healthy young women." The Journal of Nutrition 142, no. 2 (2012): 382-388.

- Ganio, Matthew S., Lawrence E. Armstrong, Douglas J. Casa, Brendon P. McDermott, Elaine C. Lee, Linda M. Yamamoto, Stefania Marzano et al. "Mild dehydration impairs cognitive performance and mood of men." British Journal of Nutrition 106, no. 10 (2011): 1535-1543.

- Kalman, Douglas S., and Anna Lepeley. "A review of hydration." Strength & Conditioning Journal 32, no. 2 (2010): 56-63.

- Leidy, Heather J., Laura C. Ortinau, Steve M. Douglas, and Heather A. Hoertel. "Beneficial effects of a higher-protein breakfast on the appetitive, hormonal, and neural signals controlling energy intake regulation in overweight/obese,"breakfast-skipping," late-adolescent girls." The American Journal of Clinical Nutrition 97, no. 4 (2013): 677-688.

- Leidy, Heather J., Mandi J. Bossingham, Richard D. Mattes, and Wayne W. Campbell. "Increased dietary protein consumed at breakfast leads to an initial and sustained feeling of fullness during energy restriction compared to other meal times." British Journal of Nutrition 101, no. 6 (2008): 798-803.

- Leidy, H. J., and E. M. Racki. "The addition of a protein-rich breakfast and its effects on acute appetite control and food intake in 'breakfast-skipping'adolescents." International Journal of Obesity 34, no. 7 (2010): 1125-1133.

- Welland, Diane, MS, RD. "Lose Weight the High-Protein Weigh." Today's Dietitian, February 2010, 34.

- Campbell, Wayne W., Marilyn C. Crim, Vernon R. Young, and William J. Evans. "Increased energy requirements and changes in body composition with resistance training in older adults." The American Journal of Clinical Nutrition 60, no. 2 (1994): 167-175.

- Pratley, R., B. Nicklas, M. Rubin, J. Miller, A. Smith, M. Smith, B. Hurley, and A. Goldberg. "Strength training increases resting metabolic rate and norepinephrine levels in healthy 50-to 65-yr-old men." Journal of Applied Physiology 76, no. 1 (1994): 133-137.

- Pikosky, Matthew A., A. Faigenbaum, Wayne Westcott, and N. Rodriguez. "The effects of resistance training on protein utilization in healthy children." Master's thesis, University of Connecticut, 2000.

- Westcott, Wayne L. "Why The Confusion on Muscle and Metabolism?."

- Paddon-Jones, Douglas, Eric Westman, Richard D. Mattes, Robert R. Wolfe, Arne Astrup, and Margriet Westerterp-Plantenga. "Protein, weight management, and satiety." The American Journal of Clinical Nutrition 87, no. 5 (2008): 1558S-1561S.

- Layman, Donald K. "Protein nutrition, meal timing, and muscle health." In Handbook of Nutrition and Food, Third Edition, pp. 861-868. CRC Press, 2013.

- "Related Topics." USDA National Nutrient Database for Standard Reference : USDA ARS. Accessed April 27, 2017. https://www.ars.usda.gov/northeast-area/beltsville-md/beltsville-human-nutrition-research-center/nutrient-data-laboratory/docs/usda-national-nutrient-database-for-standard-reference/.

- Phillips, Stuart M. "Dietary protein requirements and adaptive advantages in athletes." British Journal of Nutrition 108, no. S2 (2012): S158-S167.

- Burd, Nicholas A., Daniel WD West, Daniel R. Moore, Philip J. Atherton, Aaron W. Staples, Todd Prior, Jason E. Tang, Michael J. Rennie, Steven K. Baker, and Stuart M. Phillips. "Enhanced amino acid sensitivity of myofibrillar protein synthesis persists for up to 24 h after resistance exercise in young men." The Journal of Nutrition 141, no. 4 (2011): 568-573.

- Mamerow, Madonna M., Joni A. Mettler, Kirk L. English, Shanon L. Casperson, Emily Arentson-Lantz, Melinda Sheffield-Moore, Donald K. Layman, and Douglas Paddon-Jones. "Dietary protein distribution positively influences 24-h muscle protein synthesis in healthy adults." The Journal of Nutrition 144, no. 6 (2014): 876-880.

- Webb, Densie, PhD, RD. "Athletes and Protein Intake." Today's Dietitian, June 2014, 22.

- Thomas, D. Travis, Kelly Anne Erdman, and Louise M. Burke. "Position of the academy of nutrition and dietetics, dietitians of canada, and the american college of sports medicine: Nutrition and athletic performance." Journal of the Academy of Nutrition and Dietetics 116, no. 3 (2016): 501-528.

- Sawka, Michael N., Louise M. Burke, E. Randy Eichner, Ronald J. Maughan, Scott J. Montain, and Nina S. Stachenfeld. "American College of Sports Medicine position stand. Exercise and fluid replacement." Medicine and Science in Sports and Exercise 39, no. 2 (2007): 377-390.

- Aragon, Alan Albert, and Brad Jon Schoenfeld. "Nutrient timing revisited: is there a post-exercise anabolic window?." Journal of the International Society of Sports Nutrition 10, no. 1 (2013): 5.

- Antonio, Jose, Anya Ellerbroek, Tobin Silver, Leonel Vargas, and Corey Peacock. "The effects of a high protein diet on indices of health and body composition–a crossover trial in resistance-trained men." Journal of the International Society of Sports Nutrition 13, no. 1 (2016): 3.

- Martin, William F., Lawrence E. Armstrong, and Nancy R. Rodriguez. "Dietary protein intake and renal function." Nutrition & Metabolism 2, no. 1 (2005): 25.

Chapter 7: Buy Your Food

- Spada, Patrícia DS, Gabrielle Gianna Nunes de Souza, Giovana Vera Bortolini, João AP Henriques, and Mirian Salvador. "Antioxidant, mutagenic, and antimutagenic activity of frozen fruits." Journal of Medicinal Food 11, no. 1 (2008): 144-151.

- Thalheimer, Judith C., RD, LDNRD, LDN. "Treasures of Frozen Produce." Today's Dietitian, November 2015, 30.

- Bouzari, Ali, Dirk Holstege, and Diane M. Barrett. "Vitamin retention in eight fruits and vegetables: a comparison of refrigerated and frozen storage." Journal of Agricultural and Food Chemistry 63, no. 3 (2015): 957-962.

- "BEANS AND PEAS ARE UNIQUE FOODS." USDA ChooseMyPlate.gov. January 12, 2016. Accessed April 26, 2017. https://www.choosemyplate.gov/vegetables-beans-and-peas.

- Smith-Spangler, Crystal, Margaret L. Brandeau, Grace E. Hunter, J. Clay Bavinger, Maren Pearson, Paul J. Eschbach, Vandana Sundaram et al. "Are organic foods safer or healthier than conventional alternatives?: a systematic review." Annals of Internal Medicine 157, no. 5 (2012): 348-366.

- Thalheimer, Judith, RD, LDN. "The Organic Foods Debate — Are They Healthier Than Conventional?" Today's Dietitian, July 2013, 28.

- Yeager, David. "The Nutrition Facts Label." Today's Dietitian, July 2014, 44.

- "Latest News on Hunger in US, Africa, Asia, Global." World Hunger News. July 27, 2013. Accessed April 27, 2017. http://www.worldhunger.org/articles/Learn/world hunger facts 2002.htm.

- Giampietro, Mario. "Sustainability and technological development in agriculture." BioScience 44, no. 10 (1994): 677-689.

- Hsaio, Jennifer, and Krissy Lion. "GMOs and Pesticides: Helpful or Harmful?." Science in the News (2015).

- Wendel, JoAnna, and Jon Entine. "With 2000+ global studies affirming safety, GM foods among most analyzed subjects in science." Retrieve from https://www. geneticliteracyproject. org/2013/10/08/with-2000-global-studiesconfirming-safety-gm-foods-among-most-analyzed-subject-in-science (2013).

- Snell, Chelsea, Aude Bernheim, Jean-Baptiste Bergé, Marcel Kuntz, Gérard Pascal, Alain Paris, and Agnès E. Ricroch. "Assessment of the health impact of GM plant diets in long-term and multigenerational animal feeding trials: a literature review." Food and Chemical Toxicology 50, no. 3 (2012): 1134-1148.

- Carman, Judy A., Howard R. Vlieger, Larry J. Ver Steeg, Verlyn E. Sneller, Garth W. Robinson, Catherine A. Clinch-Jones, Julie I. Haynes, and John W. Edwards. "A long-term toxicology study on pigs fed a combined genetically modified (GM) soy and GM maize diet." J Org Syst 8, no. 1 (2013): 38-54.

- Yeager, David. "Can GMOs Harm Digestive Health? — A Controversial Animal Study Suggests GMOs May Cause Stomach Inflammation." Today's Dietitian, December 2013, 12.

- Yeager, David. "Genetically Modified Foods." Today's Dietitian, April 2014, 36.

- Thalheimer, Judith C., RD, LDN. "The Top 5 Soy Myths." Today's Dietitian, April 2014, 52. http://www.todaysdietitian.com/newarchives/040114p52.shtml.

- McCullough, M. "The Bottom Line on Soy and Breast Cancer Risk." American Cancer Society (2012).

- Center for Food Safety and Applied Nutrition. "Labeling & Nutrition - Changes to the Nutrition Facts Label." U S Food and Drug Administration Home Page. Accessed April 27, 2017. https://www.fda.gov/Food/GuidanceRegulation/GuidanceDocumentsRegulatoryInformation/LabelingNutrition/ucm385663.htm.

- Gorman, Rachael Moeller. "Flying the Coop." EatingWell, Jan. & feb. 2017, 84-92.

- Platel, Kalpana, Sushma W. Eipeson, and Krishnapura Srinivasan. "Bioaccessible mineral content of malted finger millet (Eleusine coracana), wheat (Triticum aestivum), and barley (Hordeum vulgare)." Journal of Agricultural and Food Chemistry 58, no. 13 (2010): 8100-8103.

- "Sprouted Whole Grains." Sprouted Whole Grains | The Whole Grains Council. Accessed April 27, 2017. https://wholegrainscouncil.org/whole-grains-101/whats-whole-grain-refined-grain/sprouted-whole-grains.

- Lentz, Leesha. "Whole Grains: Sprouted Grains." Today's Dietitian, June 2015, 18.

- Hoffmann, Peter R., and Marla J. Berry. "The influence of selenium on immune responses." Molecular Nutrition & Food Research 52, no. 11 (2008): 1273-1280.

- Alehagen, Urban, Peter Johansson, Mikael Björnstedt, Anders Rosén, Claes Post, and Jan Aaseth. "Relatively high mortality risk in elderly Swedish subjects with low selenium status." European Journal of Clinical Nutrition 70, no. 1 (2016): 91-96.

- Ralston, N. Selenium: The Secret That Will Change Public Perception of Seafood. Talk presented at: Academy of Nutrition and Dietetics 2016 Food and Nutrition Conference & Expo; October 16, 2016; Boston, MA.

- Ralston, NV and Raymond, NJ. (November 2010). Dietary selenium's protective effects against methylmercury toxicity. Toxicology, 278(1).

- U.S. Food and Drug Administration. (June 2014). Fish: What Pregnant Women and Parents Should Know. Draft Updated Advice by FDA and EPA.

Chapter 9: Beyond Your Food

- Mullington, Janet M., Norah S. Simpson, Hans K. Meier-Ewert, and Monika Haack. "Sleep loss and inflammation." Best Practice & Research Clinical Endocrinology & Metabolism 24, no. 5 (2010): 775-784.

- Youngstedt, Shawn D., and Christopher E. Kline. "Epidemiology of exercise and sleep." Sleep and Biological Rhythms 4, no. 3 (2006): 215-221.

- Reid, Kathryn J., Kelly Glazer Baron, Brandon Lu, Erik Naylor, Lisa Wolfe, and Phyllis C. Zee. "Aerobic exercise improves self-reported sleep and quality of life in older adults with insomnia." Sleep Medicine 11, no. 9 (2010): 934-940.

- Ussher, Michael, Amandeep K. Sampuran, Reena Doshi, Robert West, and D. Colin Drummond. "Acute effect of a brief bout of exercise on alcohol urges." Addiction 99, no. 12 (2004): 1542-1547.

- "American Heart Association Recommendations for Physical Activity in Adults." February 2014. Accessed April 27, 2017.http://www.heart.org/HEARTORG/HealthyLiving/PhysicalActivity/FitnessBasics/American-Heart-Association-Recommendations-for-Physical-Activity-in-Adults_UCM_307976_Article.jsp#.V4aD3ldNH8s.

- "American Heart Association Recommendations for Physical Activity Infographic." American Heart Association Recommendations for Physical Activity Infographic. 2016. Accessed April 27, 2017. http://www.heart.org/HEARTORG/HealthyLiving/PhysicalActivity/FitnessBasics/American-Heart-Association-Recommendations-for-Physical-Activity-Infographic_UCM_450754_SubHomePage.jsp.

- Garber, Carol Ewing, Bryan Blissmer, Michael R. Deschenes, Barry A. Franklin, Michael J. Lamonte, I-Min Lee, David C. Nieman, and David P. Swain. "Quantity and Quality of Exercise for Developing and Maintaining Cardiorespiratory, Musculoskeletal, and Neuromotor Fitness in Apparently Healthy Adults." Medicine & Science in Sports & Exercise 43, no. 7 (July 2011): 1334-359. doi:10.1249/mss.0b013e318213fefb.

- American College of Sports Medicine. "ACSM Quantity and Quality of Exercise for Developing and Maintaining Cardiorespiratory, Musculoskeletal, and Neuromotor Fitness in Apparently Healthy Adults: Guidance for Prescribing Exercise." Med Sci Sports Exerc 43, no. 7 (2011): 1334-1359.

- "How much physical activity do adults need?" Centers for Disease Control and Prevention. June 04, 2015. Accessed April 27, 2017. http://www.cdc.gov/physicalactivity/basics/adults/index.htm.

- Delavier, Frederic. Women's Strength Training Anatomy. Human Kinetics, 2003.

- Iazzetti, Giovanni, and Enrico Rigutti. Atlas of Anatomy. Taj Books Ltd, 2005. Harvard

- Clark, Micheal A., Scott Lucett, and Rodney J. Corn. NASM Essentials of Personal Fitness Training. Lippincott Williams & Wilkins, 2008.

- Folkins, Carlyle H., and Wesley E. Sime. "Physical fitness training and mental health." American Psychologist 36, no. 4 (1981): 373.

- American College of Sports Medicine. ACSM's Guidelines for Exercise Testing and Prescription. Lippincott Williams & Wilkins, 2013.

- Kondracki, Nancy L., MS, RD, LDN. "The Link Between Sleep and Weight Gain — Research Shows Poor Sleep Quality Raises Obesity and Chronic Disease Risk." Today's Dietitian, June 2012, 48.

- Morselli, Lisa L., Aurore Guyon, and Karine Spiegel. "Sleep and metabolic function." Pflügers Archiv-European Journal of Physiology 463, no. 1 (2012): 139-160.

- Chaput, J., J. Després, Claude Bouchard, and Angelo Tremblay. "The association between sleep duration and weight gain in adults: a 6-year prospective study from the Quebec Family Study." SLEEP-NEW YORK THEN WESTCHESTER- 31, no. 4 (2008): 517.

- Lyytikäinen, Peppi, Ossi Rahkonen, Eero Lahelma, and Tea Lallukka. "Association of sleep duration with weight and weight gain: a prospective follow-up study." Journal of Sleep Research 20, no. 2 (2011): 298-302.

- Stengel, Andreas, and Yvette Taché. "Ghrelin—a pleiotropic hormone secreted from endocrine X/A-like cells of the stomach." Frontiers in Neuroscience 6 (2012): 24.

- Morris, Christopher J., Sarah Fullick, Warren Gregson, Neil Clarke, Dominic Doran, Don MacLaren, and Greg Atkinson. "Paradoxical post-exercise responses of acylated ghrelin and leptin during a simulated night shift." Chronobiology International 27, no. 3 (2010): 590-605.

- Calvin, Andrew D., Rickey E. Carter, James A. Levine, and Virend K. Somers. "Abstract MP030: Insufficient Sleep Increases Caloric Intake but not Energy Expenditure." (2012): AMP030-AMP030.

- Mullington, Janet M., Norah S. Simpson, Hans K. Meier-Ewert, and Monika Haack. "Sleep loss and inflammation." Best Practice & Research Clinical Endocrinology & Metabolism 24, no. 5 (2010): 775-84. doi:10.1016/j.beem.2010.08.014.